W9-BUH-367

# Surrogate
# PARENTING

# Surrogate
# PARENTING

## AMY ZUCKERMAN OVERVOLD

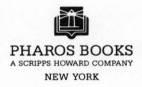

PHAROS BOOKS
A SCRIPPS HOWARD COMPANY
NEW YORK

Cover and text design: Nancy Eato

First published in 1988.

Distributed in the United States by Ballantine Books, a division of Random House Inc., and in Canada by Random House of Canada, Ltd.

Library of Congress Cataloging-in-Publication Data

Overvold, Amy Zuckerman.
Surrogate parenting.

Includes index.
1. Surrogate mothers—United States. 2. Artificial insemination, Human—Moral and ethical aspects. 3. Artificial insemination, Human—Law and legislation—United States. 4. Fertilization in vitro, Human—Moral and ethical aspects. 5. Fertilization in vitro, Human—Moral and ethical aspects. 6. Fertilization in vitro, Human—United States—Directories.
I. Title.
HQ759.5.093    1988    306.8'743    87-50915

Pharos Books ISBN: 0-88687-328-2
Ballantine ISBN: 0-345-35225-4

Printed in the United States of America

Pharos Books
A Scripps Howard Company
200 Park Avenue
New York, NY 10166

10   9   8   7   6   5   4   3   2   1

To my mother, Florence Margolis Zuckerman, who was
the first to show me the music in words.

# ACKNOWLEDGEMENTS

A very special thanks to all the clinic directors, couples, and surrogates nationwide who assisted in the preparation of this book, especially Laraine Shore-Suslowitz, Hilary Hanafin, Lyn Brown, and Beth Bacon.

Thanks also to the following people who gave encouragement, advice, and support: my husband, Gary Overvold, Robert Cormier, B. A. King, Kenneth Davis, Thomas Goethals, Charles Blinderman, Angela Dorenkamp, Beranrd Gotfryd, Alan Lupo, B. Michael Zuckerman, Kathleen Shaw, Geraldine Collier, Betty Ann Caputo, Betty Lewis, Danna Peterson, Polly Pruneau, Peter Longo, Ethel Theodore, Marjorie Waterbrook, Ann Mancini, Kathy Pierce, my agent Anita Diamant, and my editor Hana Umlauf Lane.

And a final thanks to my "surrogate" children, Geoffrey, Kristi and Heidi Overvold, who served as inspiration for this book.

# CONTENTS

# Introduction

Surrogate parenting was still in its infancy when I began researching the subject in December 1985. Although surrogate parenting clinics had been in existence nationwide for almost ten years, the procedure was relatively obscure. Very little had been published on surrogacy and, certainly, no one had anticipated a "Baby M" custody battle.

At the time I was a reporter for the life-style section of *The Evening Gazette* in Worcester, Massachusetts. One day that December a call came into the office from a man who said he and his wife had hired a surrogate mother to bear their child. The call spoke to me. As a childless woman in my thirties, I knew I could very well face fertility problems. I, too, could be a candidate for surrogate parenting. In the week before meeting Glenn and Linda McRobbie, I wondered what it would be like to be a prospective parent awaiting the birth of my child via a stranger in another state. And what would induce me to be that other woman, the woman who was carrying a child for strangers?

Listening to the McRobbies' story of woe—a story of miscarriages, cancer, failed adoption attempts, psychological trauma, and misery—raised many more questions. Should there have been a price tag on the process? How would they explain their child's birth to him or her? How could the surrogate give up the child she had carried for nine months? Was $10,000 sufficient payment for such a service?

Moreover, who would take such an immense legal risk? In Massachusetts, as in many states, surrogate parenting was not yet recognized in the courts. If a Massachusetts surrogate were to break her contract and refuse to release the child—as would happen in New Jersey a few months later—there was no precedent to determine whether the court would throw the case out without a hearing, grant the surrogate the child, or force her to hand it over to the couple who had contracted for its birth. The smattering of cases across the country in which surrogate parenting contracts had been challenged were not conclusive. In her 1984 book *New Conceptions*—a handbook for people interested in pioneer reproductive techniques—Lori Andrews, a lawyer for the American Bar Association in Chicago, wrote that surrogacy without legal protection "is a legally risky procedure. We need laws that clarify the rights and responsibilities of the parties involved."

The McRobbies, an affable, average American couple, were well aware of the risks when they first contacted a New England surrogate parenting center in December 1984. But they didn't care. They desperately wanted a child, and there wasn't much they hadn't confronted in their pursuit of this dream. If nature had conspired against them, they would become reproductive pioneers.

Surrogacy proved rewarding for the McRobbies. Unlike those who have faced problems with surrogates, paternity laws, or children born handicapped, the case of the McRobbies was a "normal" one that produced a healthy, thriving baby. How they got to that point, though, is a story filled with psychological anguish, with doubts, anxiety and financial difficulties, as well as joy. But the story does not end here. There are potential problems down the road. Like all couples who have children via surrogate mother, the McRobbies have the difficult task of one day explaining to their son how he was conceived. They must decide whether to continue a relationship with the surrogate and what to tell their son about the woman's daughter, who is legally his half sister. There is also the worry of how others will react if they learn about their son's background. And then there are the more general questions—the moral, ethical issues. What does surrogacy mean? What impact will it have on society in the future? Is it wrong to bring children into the world in this manner? Is surrogate parenting playing God, or is it no different from adoption?

These questions have sparked heated discussion and controversy among experts in reproductive science. In July 1982 British scientists, physicians, and numerous others in related fields joined forces to study the implications of various new reproductive methods. The Wornack report, the result of their study, was published after the birth of the first child via in vitro fertilization in 1978. The report stated that "events were moving too fast for their implications to be assimilated" and that there had to be "some barriers that are not to be crossed, some limits fixed, beyond which people must not be allowed to go." One of the methods discussed in the report was surrogate parenting. Those who contributed to the chapter on surrogacy were divided on the issue of whether it should be allowed as a means of combating infertility or banned. The majority not only recommended that the process be banned, but that operating a surrogate parenting clinic be made a criminal act in England. The reasons given for such an extreme recommendation would not surprise people, like the McRobbies, who have lived through surrogacy. According to the Wornack report, surrogacy raises too many psychological and legal questions whose outcome cannot yet be determined. Among these is the question of whether surrogate parenting does not confuse the issue of motherhood and may not be a form of exploiting one human being for the benefit of others. For example, should the courts recognize the genetic mother—in the McRobbies' case Helen, the surrogate—or the adoptive mother, which Linda McRobbie would become? Among the authors of the Wornack report who favored banning surrogacy there was some feeling that it should be provided on a limited, nonprofit basis. But even that proposal was deemed unworkable because it would probably encourage the growth of the procedure.

In the years since the publication of the Wornack report, American fertility experts and the Catholic church have joined the chorus of those concerned about surrogate parenting. When the American Fertility Society convened to discuss the phenomenon in September 1986, the ten thousand doctors, scientists, and specialists on fertility who make up the organization expressed "serious ethical reservations" about surrogacy and called for "intensive scrutiny" of the practice because of legal and ethical concerns, and because so little is known about the physical and psychological effects on those involved. That same month the National [American] Committee for Adoption called for a ban on surrogate parenting. Committee President William Pierce said, "It commercializes a very private thing. It should not take place at all." (*Newsweek*, September 22, 1986.)

Despite the predominant chorus of naysayers, it should also be noted that there are experts who regard surrogate parenting in a different light and who, out of compassion for infertile couples like the McRobbies, do not favor banning the process. There were members of the British medical/scientific establishment who filed a dissenting report to the surrogate parenting chapter of the Wornack report. These experts understood the risks involved in the process but felt that some risk was an unavoidable aspect of helping infer-

tile couples. They recommended that the process be legalized and all surrogate parenting clinics licensed. The clinics
would then be categorized as nonprofit to avoid exploitation
of both the surrogates and the participating couples. They
felt it would be unfortunate to ban surrogate parenting
while "public opinion is not yet fully formed on the question of surrogacy." They go on to say: "Thus we think it is
too early to take a final decision one way or the other. We
wish to have the opportunity in the next few years to see
what the demand is, whether an agency is prepared to come
forward to satisfy it, and whether the consequences are generally acceptable or not. We simply ask that the door be left
slightly ajar so that surrogacy can be more effectively
assessed."

The McRobbies have a baby today because the courts and
state legislatures in the United States kept that door ajar.
They would like to see surrogacy regulated. They would like
to see the adoptive mother granted legal status from the
time of conception, and they would have liked to have suffered less emotional anguish during the surrogate parenting
process. But they would hate not to have their son.

I, too, would leave the door open for couples like the
McRobbies. Despite the controversy inherent in the procedure, surrogate parenting is here to stay. The "Baby M" rul-
ing made it clear that at least one judge in one state considered a surrogate parenting contract binding and the process
legitimate. In the wake of that case, surrogate parenting
clinics nationwide were swamped with inquiries from both
prospective surrogates and couples. Rather than turn people
off the surrogate parenting process, the New Jersey court
battle made thousands of infertile couples aware of its existence. The Catholic church and the writers of the Wornack
report may rail against the practice and state legislatures
may attempt to ban it, but I doubt that church bans or legislation will have much impact on surrogate parenting. Infertile couples have already demonstrated to what extraordi-

nary lengths they will go to have a child. Outlawing surrogate parenting would simply drive the process underground.

Surrogate parenting, not yet legalized in most states at the time of this writing, continues to operate half in the shadows and half in the light of our consciousness. To allow it to remain in the shadows will mean more "Baby M" cases, more harm to innocent people. After talking with surrogates, couples, clinic directors, and psychologists nationwide, it became clear that some sort of regulation of the process is needed. In fact, a majority of those already involved in surrogate parenting favor legalization of the procedure, licensing of clinics, and standardization of surrogate parenting practices. These people would like to see surrogate parenting brought into the mainstream where it can gain respectablity and acceptance. They realize that it will be much easier on the children involved if society regards surrogate parenting as it does adoption. They also realize that this respectability and acceptance will not exist while anyone can open up a surrogate parenting clinic; while screening of surrogates and couples is haphazard at best; and while clinics and centers can reap huge profits based on the misfortune of others. Furthermore, surrogate parenting will not gain general acceptance until clinic directors drop their bunker mentality and realize that the procedure as now practiced is imperfect. Attacks on the process seem to have blinded many in the field to the emotional problems surrogate parenting can produce including marital stress, postpartum adjustment difficulties for the surrogate, and future emotional issues for the child. Surrogate parenting clinics and centers have a responsibility to assist their clients through a potentially difficult period. Unfortunately, what some clinics pass off as counseling really amounts to indoctrination in favor of surrogacy.

With all my sympathy for surrogate parenting, I am open to the notion that even a "normal" surrogacy case can produce thorny emotional issues for all parties concerned. I have also learned that education and counseling would go a long way toward alleviating many of the problems couples and surrogates have encountered. My aim in writing this book is to offer a source of general information on surrogate parenting and a psychological and ethical guide to those who may be tempted to seek out this method.

Those who are interested in exploring this procedure should ask two questions of themselves before making a commitment: Is surrogate parenting ethically right for me? Do I understand and am I prepared to accept the predictable difficulties the procedure entails? The surrogates and couples who passed over this crucial questioning stage—the Mary Beth Whiteheads, for example—have become the stuff of headlines. Surrogate parenting can work for those who enter the process with the full awareness that their actions will have wide-ranging consequences. I offer this inside look at the procedure with the hope that it will make for intelligent and informed decisions that lead to sound, healthy surrogate parenting experiences.

# 1

## THE COUPLES

# 1 | The Birth: What Surrogate Parenting is All About

Bernard Glennon McRobbie came into the world the usual way at 2:01 A.M. on April 9, 1986. His birth was a quick one. So quick, in fact, that there was no immediate way to notify his parents that the surrogate mother—the woman with whom they had contracted to bear their child—was in labor. Because the hospital switchboard was shut down during the early morning hours, the McRobbies didn't learn of their son's birth until five and a half hours after the fact. And because they lived in another state some one hundred miles from the hospital, they did not see their son for another four hours after that.

When that long-awaited call finally came at 7:30 A.M. on April 9, Linda McRobbie was downstairs making a cup of coffee in the kitchen of their Massachusetts home, and her husband, Glenn, was upstairs dressing. Except for the tension both were feeling because Bernie was almost three weeks late, April 9 was just another workday. Glenn was getting ready to go to his job at a bank in a nearby community, and Linda was preparing to spend the day on house plans for a client.

Neither of the McRobbies had slept much since the third week of March, the baby's revised due date. Ultrasound had revealed his sex and the fact that he appeared to be a large baby. Consequently, the surrogate's obstetrician had pushed back the due date from March 30 to March 23. But the twenty-third had come and gone, then the thirtieth, April Fool's Day, and another week after that. Emotions were strained, nerves unbearably taut. After waiting seven years to have a child, the McRobbies found it incredible that they should have to wait another day. And then, always in the back of their minds, was that horrendous question. Would the surrogate, Helen, give up the child as agreed?

But when Monday, April 7 rolled around—another tense weekend of fruitless waiting had passed—the McRobbies had begun to relax. It seemed that this baby didn't want to be born. There was no use tossing and turning every night in anticipation of that crucial phone call. The people at the New England clinic where the McRobbies had contracted to have a child reported that the baby was still active. There would not be a decision on whether to induce labor until Thursday of that week—Thursday, April 10.

Little wonder, then, that the news of the birth caught the McRobbies so completely off guard that they were unable to fully comprehend what had happened. According to the arrangement, the clinic was to contact the McRobbies when the surrogate mother went into labor. The McRobbies would then drive to the designated hospital in New York state to be on hand for the birth. The news they were awaiting that morning was that labor had begun. Realizing that their son was already born, Glenn and Linda were so exhilarated and relieved that they hardly knew what to say or feel.

'It's a boy,' the woman from the clinic calmly told me," Linda McRobbie later related. "I remember thinking how ridiculous this was, because we already knew it was going to be a boy. It wasn't until she started telling me things like he weighed in at 6.1 pounds that I realized Bernie was born."

Linda remembers half listening to the details of the birth and hurriedly making a mental list of things to be accomplished before their departure. From the clinic she learned that the surrogate had seen the obstetrician on the previous afternoon and he had taken measures to induce labor. Cramping started at around 10:30 that night. By the time Helen arrived at the hospital, labor was well under way and birth appeared imminent. What ensued was a race to get Helen to the delivery room before the birth could take place. Attendants rolled her down hospital corridors on a table as the doctor raced to catch up, literally throwing on a surgical gown as he ran.

Helen later told the clinic there was one big contraction, and Bernie was born. He entered the world with his hands held over his head—"ready to launch a dunk shot," said Glenn, an avid basketball fan—and sucking his lower lip from hunger. The placenta had collapsed during the weeks before his birth, forcing the fetus to live off his own fat. That was a major reason he was smaller than expected.

As soon as Linda hung up the phone, she began to worry. The contact with her baby had been severed with the phone connection. Instead of being on hand for the birth, as had been planned, she was miles away and the baby was alone with its biological mother nearby. Linda greatly feared the power of the surrogate—the power of the biological mother. She was afraid the baby that was to be hers via adoption would start bonding with the surrogate. Someone had told her that newborns can smell their mother's milk, and this thought—true or false—raced through her mind. In her haste to get going, she tripped on her nightgown on the way up the stairs to the bedroom. They weren't even packed. Time was awasting, she told herself.

Glenn, who was upstairs when Linda took the call, heard her screaming and panicked. Someone had died, he thought, or the field outside the house was on fire. Gradually, as if the whole scene was being played out in slow motion, he began to comprehend what his wife was screaming. "We have a son," he said to himself. "The baby is born."

In those first few moments of dawning realization, Glenn discovered that he was as shocked as he was excited. He couldn't believe the baby was already born. It wasn't supposed to happen that way. His first reaction was to run around in fifty directions and do nothing. His only thought was to get to the hospital right away and make sure the surrogate released the baby. But calls had to be made—to the people who were checking on the house and to his office. All the preparations took a little more than an hour; but that was an eternity under the circumstances. It was 8:45 before Glenn backed the car out of the garage and the McRobbies headed down the winding country road that took them to the highway.

To Linda everything seemed surreal—the news, all the emotions, and then Glenn flying down the highway, eating up the miles that separated them from their son. They drove in a daze of exhaustion and anxiety, and with good reason. This was no average trip to the hospital to pick up your newborn. This wasn't even comparable to going to an adoption agency for a child. When the McRobbies left their house early that morning in April they faced a host of unknowns. When would they see the baby? When would the relinquishment proceedings take place? Would the surrogate give up the child? Even if she agreed to give up the child, would she insist on spending a lot of time with the baby during her hospital convalescence? Would she be able to break the emotional and psychological ties that bind?

In the month or so before the birth, Linda had spent countless hours worrying about these questions. And she had a few fears of her own. Would she be able to bond with an infant she had not carried? Would she have to fight for access to her baby in the hospital? Would the surrogate, as the biological mother, usurp her maternal role? As the process neared a climax, the McRobbies became more and more conscious of the fact that surrogate parenting was still highly experimental. Despite lengthy contracts with the clinic and the surrogate, there was no guarantee that a Massachusetts court of law would uphold their claim. There was no guarantee that the surrogate would relinquish their child and no guarantee that a court of law would force her to do so if she reneged.

Little wonder, then, that Glenn was burning up those miles. He wanted to be with his son, not watching the road signs fly by on the Massachusetts Turnpike. As he drove, Glenn rehearsed in his mind what he would do if they were greeted with the news that Helen refused to abide by her part of the contract. As it turned out, no one greeted the McRobbies when they finally reached the hospital at 11:15 A.M. What they found was a large brick, institutional sort of place. "The type that looms up at you with wings all over the place—a really big medical center," Glenn recalled. When they entered the lobby by a side entrance they found a long, narrow room with ugly carpeting and wood paneling, almost like a library. Glenn found the hospital's appearance somehow comforting. He was glad it wasn't intimidating with gleaming antiseptic white walls.

The McRobbies happened to arrive at a moment when activity in the lobby was at its peak. Nurses, doctors, orderlies, and visitors seemed to be coming out of every nook and cranny. Dazed by the confusion, they managed to get directions to the nursery from the front desk. The instructions sent them down a long corridor where no elevators were to be found. After some searching, they discovered the elevators only to find that only one was in service. The wait for the elevator seemed interminable to Glenn, whose patience had worn thin. To have to wait this long to see his newborn son seemed particularly cruel. Being forced to stop at each floor on the way up to the nursery seemed more cruel still.

Finally, they reached the right floor, but no nursery was in sight.

A nurse sent the McRobbies along a circuitous route that brought them back above the lobby. They eventually found the place, but neither the head nurse of the maternity ward nor a hospital coordinator was there to greet them as had been planned. No one was there. No one, that is, except their little son. As they watched through the nursery window they could see Bernie being fed by a nurse. They wanted to reach through the glass and grab the baby from her. But for the time being they had to be content with watching. The relinquishment proceedings came first. To Glenn this moment was one of the worst in the entire surrogacy process. Knowing they couldn't cuddle their child, that legalities were a priority, put a damper on the thrill of seeing his son for the first time. Linda had similar feelings about the situation. It was as if someone was dangling a carrot from a stick.

The sight of Elaine Silver, director of the clinic, coming down the corridor with a dour-looking man—the surrogate's lawyer, as it turned out—cut short their time at the nursery window. This wasn't the welcoming party the McRobbies had expected. Neither the lawyer nor Elaine was smiling. They panicked. They had no idea the lawyer came with Helen's word to release Bernie to them. What if they never experienced the joy of holding him in their arms? Luckily, no such trauma took place. Because this was New York State, release of custody to Glenn could take place immediately, right on the premises. If the birth had taken place in Massachusetts, there would have been a four-day wait to verify paternity—that much longer to worry.

Elaine beckoned the three of them into a small office opposite the nursery. As she did so, she casually noted that Helen was approaching the nursery window where the McRobbies had been standing minutes before. Because the McRobbies had chosen to avoid contact with their surrogate, there was a moment of panic. Glenn was able to duck around a corner, but Linda, who was too stunned to move, caught a glimpse of the other woman's back.

The experience might have been more unsettling if they hadn't immediately plunged into the legal issues. There was a tense moment when the lawyer left to get the surrogate's signature and another when Linda added her signature to the relinquishment papers. As she took up the pen, she realized that after all the months of waiting, the months of worry, she was finally a step closer to being Bernie's legal mother. Under Massachusetts law, the state where Bernie would live, the adoption would not take place for six months. As Linda and Glenn went through the motions that would legally release Bernie into their custody, adoption seemed a distant, somewhat irrelevant proposition. They were in the hospital, the baby was theirs and with Glenn the biological father, the adoption seemed certain. They had no time or inclination to dwell on any negative consequences. The only thing that mattered was seeing Bernie, holding him, touching him.

The relinquishment process took about an hour. By then it was 12:15. For the first time in months the McRobbies began to relax. The moment was especially blissful for Linda. Although she and Glenn had signed a contract with the clinic and the surrogate had done the same months earlier, the initial legal work had provided scant security during those horrendous weeks leading up to the birth. Throughout Helen's pregnancy, the McRobbies lived with the fear that they would have to wage a custody battle of the kind that would rock the nation several months later when surrogate Mary Beth Whitehead refused to give up "Baby M." If things came to such a showdown, neither Glenn nor Linda was certain the contract "would do a darn bit of good."

Signing the relinquishment papers would at least give them a little more security in their newly acquired parental role. And once the last signature was in place, the McRobbies would finally be free to visit with their son for a lifetime.

They entered the gold-toned nursery and found two sets of hospital cribs divided by a work area for the staff. A nurse led them to the crib where their son was sleeping. To facilitate Linda's bonding with Bernie, it had been prearranged that she would be the first to hold him. What she felt was disbelief, coupled with fear, at the thought that this tiny, six-pound creature was truly hers. All those years of trying to become pregnant, of suffering uterine cancer, and then watching her father die of cancer before Bernie had even been conceived—all that pain and suffering disappeared as she held the little bundle in her arms. Linda couldn't get over how small he was, how fragile, and how damaged his face was by the birth.

The relief of having all those papers signed at last and the sight of the baby's "smooshed" face, as she kept calling it, masked the intense emotion Linda felt. She was more scared than excited, she realized. But, by the time she held her son again, she felt her fears beginning to evaporate. Maternal instinct began to hold sway. Bernie was her baby now. A feeling of intense protectiveness came over Linda, who said, "If anyone had tried to take him away, I would have attacked them. I was surprised at how I felt."

Glenn was equally afraid and elated. He couldn't get over the fact that he was finally a father. "I couldn't believe how little he was," he recalled. "I felt the bonding immediately. I felt protective. I had worried about his health and whether the surrogate would release him. Seeing that lawyer was like a knife in my heart. I was really frightened for a few minutes."

Reluctantly, the McRobbies left their son in the nursery to join Elaine for lunch in the hospital's cafeteria. Over their light fare, they learned that the surrogate's lawyer had been impressed with them and had related his positive feelings to his client. She in turn had expressed a desire to meet them.

Glenn immediately turned to Linda. He felt the decision was hers to make.

Before arriving at the hospital Linda would have said no to all contact with Helen. For a while, during the early stages of the pregnancy, she had been tempted to assist at the birth in order to gain immediate access to the baby. But the physical distance between the McRobbies' house and the hospital made it unlikely they could arrive in time to be present at the birth. And then she had qualms about meeting this woman. She had been told repeatedly how much they looked alike, and that was very important to Linda. What if she was disappointed? What if they didn't resemble each other at all? What if they became emotionally attached to each other? Would Linda be able to go along with this woman giving up the baby? Given all the latent psychological issues surrounding her relationship with the surrogate, Linda and Glenn decided that anonymity was preferable.

Anonymity in the true sense of the word, however, was pretty much tossed to the wind once the surrogate became pregnant via artificial insemination using Glenn's sperm. Although the McRobbies did not have the surrogate's address, they knew her name and had often sent her letters through the clinic. Gifts had been sent on special occasions, such as Christmas, for both the surrogate and her little girl. The surrogate had sent letters in return and had requested pictures of the McRobbies to show her daughter. As the pregnancy wore on and the attention of the clinic shifted from the McRobbies to the surrogate's progress, the McRobbies had sometimes found themselves privy to more information about the surrogate than they cared to know. They felt it was hard enough for them to juggle their own emotional needs without worrying about Helen and the problems the pregnancy was creating with her boyfriend and her daughter. They didn't want the guilt, and, moreover, they felt they didn't deserve it.

Linda had been particularly adamant that the surrogacy

be a business transaction. She was having a hard enough time coping with the anxiety and tension of the situation without suffering for the other woman as well. At no time did she feel the need to make the process businesslike as much as during those first hours in the hospital when the surrogate—the woman who had brought them so much joy and could bring them so much sorrow—lurked nearby. Linda wanted to tell her, "You opted to do this; now he's mine. Let's close the chapter."

But nothing in life, she had discovered, was that easy. She and Glenn soon came to see that surrogate parenting was a business transaction only in the sense that money changes hands and contracts are signed. But neither of them was prepared for the emotional roller coaster it represented—and certainly not in the hospital at a time when their feelings should have been those of unadulterated bliss and joy. The knowledge that the other woman was up and mobile, and very keen on visiting Bernie, was upsetting. It also meant that an encounter with Helen might be a distinct possibility.

In the end it was that first sight of the baby's "crushed" face that made it imperative for Linda to find out what this woman looked like. The first meeting between the McRobbies and their surrogate mother took place a little before 2:00 P.M. in the surrogate's hospital room. The McRobbies found her lying in bed in an old room with high ceilings, two-tone institutional green walls, exposed heating, and drab draperies. Her pleasant appearance and kind demeanor made up for the less than cheerful setting and immediately put the McRobbies at ease. Both Linda and Glenn were relieved to find that their child's biological mother, though somewhat nondescript, did have regular features. Elaine had told them that she had no chin, and Linda, having had no experience with newborns, had felt a moment of panic when the baby, too, appeared to have no chin. Both she and Linda had the same light coloring, but Linda felt that the resemblance ended there.

All of these observations were made in a flash as they entered the room. Everyone in the room seemed to be affected
in their own way. Without thinking, Linda approached the
woman in bed and gave her a hug and a kiss, along with the
presents they had brought for her. Her heart was pounding
a million times a minute. "The first thing I said to her was
that I wanted Glenn to take off his shoes so she could see
where Bernie got his feet. That's how nervous I was, " Linda
recalled.

Glenn was overwhelmed by the strangeness of meeting
the woman who had been inseminated with his sperm—a
woman he had never seen or touched or talked with until
this moment, and yet who had joined with him to create a
life. Reflecting on the absurdity of the insemination process,
he later said, "The closest I got to her before was when she
was on the second floor of the doctor's building ovulating
and I was on the first floor with an empty jar in my hand."
Once the awkwardness had worn off and they compared
notes on the pregnancy and birth, he was relieved. Glenn
could see that the woman was not educated but had "a good
head on her shoulders." As the conversation wore on he
tried to impress upon her their deep appreciation for what
she had done for them. And as he did so, he knew that
words could never convey the full extent of his gratitude.

Helen, it turned out, had an agenda of her own. She was
hoping the McRobbies would be good parents for Bernie—
the sort of people who really cared about children and
would take pains to give him a good upbringing. Although
she had no physical problems associated with the birth, the
experience had left its psychic scars. Meeting the McRobbies
made Helen feel better about everything. She felt she could
turn Bernie over to them without undue concern. As they
turned to leave she called out to them, "I'm glad you're
happy."

The next twenty-four hours proved to be a crazy whirl for
the McRobbies. Apart from eating and sleeping, they spent

all their time at the hospital with their son. The idea was for them to have a chance to learn to care for the baby before bringing him home. They did learn some things—how to force-feed him, for example—but the nursing staff was not particularly helpful. The McRobbies felt that some of the older nurses disapproved of them and what they had done. Some of them acted as if the McRobbies were usurping what they saw as the rightful role of the biological mother to be alone with her baby. The nurses' negative attitudes made the McRobbies anxious about leaving Bernie alone in the hospital that night. Would the baby be all right? How often did the surrogate visit him? Fortunately, they were so exhausted from the excitement and tension that they both sank into deep sleep by 9:00 P.M.

When they awoke in the morning, Glenn and Linda were determined to be back at the hospital with their son as soon as they could shower and throw on some clothes. Linda was particularly anxious because she couldn't overcome her concern that some bonding might take place between the surrogate and Bernie. Meeting Helen had helped, but it didn't totally alleviate the problem. Helen was still in the hospital, and she still had access to the baby.

It wasn't that Linda was unsympathetic to the surrogate mother who had borne their baby. As a woman who had desperately wanted to have a child of her own, she understood Helen's anguish at having to relinquish the child. It was all very real to her. So real, in fact, that Linda needed to tune out the surrogate and her situation. She did so by concentrating on the positive things, the successful relinquishment and, most of all, on the baby. But it wasn't easy to tune out the message the surrogate brought with her when they met for a second time the following day.

The McRobbies were inside holding Bernie—Linda admits to "hogging him"—when they caught sight of Helen passing by. When she looked slightly embarrassed to see them, Glenn ran after her to reassure her that she was welcome. Despite the awkwardness she agreed, and they gathered together in a small room off the main nursery. Although Linda felt more relaxed than she had the day before, she couldn't prevent herself from hovering over the baby the entire time the surrogate was near. Later she confessed to admiring Helen's restraint. She could see that the other woman was dying to hold the baby, but she kept her distance. They talked about the surrogate's five-year-old daughter and the difficulty she had accepting the fact that her mother wouldn't be bringing a little brother or sister home with her. The girl had put up such a fuss that Helen refused to let her come to the hospital to visit. Helen confided to the McRobbies that she wasn't sure how her daughter would react to losing her half brother.

The meeting lasted only a few minutes, but the impact was indelible. When Helen stood to leave, she became extremely emotional. Teary-eyed, she kissed the baby on his head and said, "Good-bye, Bernie." Before leaving the room, however, she handed the McRobbies an envelope that she asked them to give to Bernie when they felt it was appropriate. As the surrogate mother walked away from the baby she had carried for so many months, Linda could have wept. Even tougher for her and Glenn, though, was absorbing the contents of the envelope. Inside was a note to Linda and Glenn dated April 10, 1986. "Can you please keep this for Bernie to let him know just how much I do love him?" Helen had written. Included was a card showing a baby cradled in the palm of a large hand. Inscribed below was a verse from Isaiah: "See! I will not forget you. For I have carved you on the palm of my hand."

If ever the McRobbies' joy took a back seat, it was during the moment they read Helen's note. She had left them no choice but to feel her pain. Moreover, for the first time, they were forced to confront the issue of what to tell their son about his conception when he reached the age of understanding. Linda's first reaction was one of dismay. "I felt badly that she wrote it, and angry," she said. "But I have to understand her feelings." Glenn added, "It was a heartbreaker."

Linda agreed, but the note and card from the surrogate made her more determined than ever to break the connection between them. Reluctantly, she also agreed to Helen's request for a photograph of Bernie's nursery and a picture of the little boy when he was a year old. These were magnanimous gestures on Linda's part, for the threat of the biological mother was very real to her. It was with relief that the McRobbies drove off with Bernie midmorning on Friday, April 11. But the reminder of Helen's connection to Bernie lingered. On their way out of the hospital they were handed some gifts Helen's daughter had sent for the baby.

The McRobbies know that one day they will want to tell Bernie about his biological mother and half sister—the other people who are connected to him by birth. Neither of them is happy about the prospect, but both understand the necessity. "You can't hide it," Glenn said, nuzzling his little son's nose. "He'll probably be told starting at an age when he's too young to understand, so it will always be part of his knowledge. We figure he'll want to know someday."

# 2 | The Nightmare Years: Why a Couple Turns to Surrogacy

When Glenn and Linda first started dating in the winter of 1979 both worked for a large western Massachusetts insurance company. At best they were passing acquaintances—two people who occasionally exchanged a few words in the corridor. Glenn thought Linda was pretty attractive, but he assumed she had a boyfriend. A colleague informed him otherwise and encouraged him to ask her out. He took her to dinner. Linda found him "serious, conservative, soft-spoken, kind, and family oriented." But she was so afraid of falling in love with him, of reviving that dream of marriage and family that her divorce had destroyed, that she hardly looked at Glenn all evening. The next day friends asked her what Glenn looked like, and she couldn't tell them. She had spent most of the evening staring into her plate.

By the third date, though, Glenn and Linda were wildly euphoric about each other. They seemed to know that marriage was in their future. Glenn made Linda feel confident and secure. "We had the same goals," she pointed out. "We always thought alike." Glenn put it similarly: "We were both looking for the same thing. We're both hardworking, we like sharing around the household. And, of course, we were attracted to each other."

The main goal they shared, however, was a desire for children. That was a given, something they didn't need to discuss much in the course of their whirlwind romance. Somehow it was understood that marriage for them meant a family. From childhood both McRobbies had individually dreamed of marriage and children. But early marriages for each had led to divorce, and they had both spent their twenties as single people. By the time they started to date, they had pretty much adjusted to—if not accepted—their single status. Both were thirty. Parenthood seemed a remote possibility.

For Linda there was always the unspoken fear that she might be infertile. It was a concern she chose not to share with Glenn during those heady, bubbly days of their early romance. It wasn't something she particularly wanted to dwell on herself. She wanted to savor the fantasy of a life with Glenn and their children. After all she had suffered during her single years, she felt she deserved a little happiness. For Linda, happiness was a precious commodity, something that had been in scant supply when she was a child growing up. She was an only child, the product of a tempestuous marriage. Personality differences had been the cause of her parents' violent, nightly clashes. Lying in her bedroom, cringing at the angry voices in the next room, Linda had escaped time and again into her fantasy of a happy, warm family life.

Not long after leaving home to go to college, Linda met her first husband, Garrett. In retrospect, she thinks they were a mismatch. She craved stability and her young fiance was a roamer. Right after proposing, Garrett joined the Marine Corps and was shipped out for basic training. When he returned, life proved less than harmonious. He and Linda were divorced several years later. During her brief marriage Linda had given up on her goal of having a family. Although she believes she was pregnant and miscarried at least once, she never bothered to find out what had happened medically. At the time, it didn't seem to matter. She later realized that the marriage lacked the trust and stability necessary for raising children.

When she and Garrett were divorced, Linda had no choice but to postpone having a family. "Friends were having children, but I put that at the back of my mind and went on with life," she recalled. "I became career-oriented and my career took off." Over a period of seven years, Linda advanced from a draftsman to her present status of a self-taught interior designer. Unfortunately, her personal life wasn't as successful as her career. She was engaged three times after her divorce only to have each of the relationships fall apart. What these men had in common was a macho quality that Linda found appealing in small doses. None of them ever talked about having a family.

Glenn was different. Open, warm, enthusiastic, he could be supportive and caring in a way that Linda had never experienced in a man of her own age. For Glenn, establishing a loving environment for raising a family was the natural thing to do. It was the way he had been raised. Born into a comfortable, middle-class family straight out of "Leave It to Beaver," Glenn's was an ideal childhood: "We had no idea of poverty," he said, reminiscing. "We had a warm, stable household. I was so happy growing up that when I went to bed at night I couldn't wait to get up the next morning to see what the day would bring."

An extremely active, imaginative child, Glenn soon became aware that the adult world was different. At puberty he already longed to return to childhood. That's when he decided that he would have three children when he grew up—just like his parents—so he could relive his own youth. But the rebellious 1960s proved trying for an adolescent with such traditional values. While other teenagers of his generation were experimenting with drugs and sex, Glenn spent his high school years on the basketball court or the baseball field. He didn't find himself until he transferred from Tufts University to Florida Southern, a conservative school that offered him a full basketball scholarship. There he met his future wife, Mary. They had a romance filled with innocent fun and were married two weeks after graduation in 1971. The marriage seemed to work just fine as long as Glenn kept the real world from intruding. That meant no talk of children and no talk of the future.

Although Glenn still longed for a family, he held his tongue around his young wife. He could see that she was having trouble reconciling her marriage with the demands of a career. Moreover, from 1973 to 1976 he worked during the day and earned a master's degree in finance at night. Starting a family just wasn't practical. As the years passed, though, no time seemed right for Mary. She became increasingly upset whenever pregnancy was mentioned. Her job was becoming more and more important, and by the time she was twenty-four she began to make it known that she didn't want children. Then she decided to leave and do her own thing.

Glenn took a job at the same western Massachusetts insurance company where he would eventually meet Linda and settled down to an uneasy bachelorhood. When he wasn't worrying about whether he would ever be a father, he worried about being an old parent. In Linda he not only found a playmate but someone with whom he could share his future. They were engaged several months after their first date and started working on getting pregnant almost immediately. They were both prepared for a long wait. It took a few weeks. They moved the wedding date back from January of 1980 to October 19, 1979.

Linda, who felt over the hill at thirty, was thrilled with the news. Glenn took it all in stride. He had simply assumed that nature would take its course. They had been trying, hadn't they? But things weren't that simple. Linda began suffering lower back pain that was so unbearable she found it difficult to stand. Before long, she had to stop wearing high-heeled shoes. Wedding plans distracted her from the physical discomfort. But the day of the wedding she was in such agony that she had to wear flat shoes to the ceremony, which was held in a pretty Congregational church near their new home. Only the prospect of marrying Glenn and the excitement of the moment got her through the short service and the cake cutting and toasts back at the house.

The wedding took place at 7:00 P.M. By 9:00 Linda and Glenn were in bed playing cribbage. Linda had begun hemorrhaging when they returned from the church. The next morning the bleeding was serious enough to warrant hospitalization. Lying in a hospital bed, depressed and terrified at what was happening, Linda remembered the nagging fears of her first pregnancy—that inner, gut feeling that she would have a hard time having a baby. The doctor confirmed what she had already suspected; she was miscarrying.

Linda was released from the hospital with the warning that she stay in touch with a gynecologist. The gynecologist in turn did an ultrasound. The results, which arrived several weeks later, were so ominous that immediate hospitalization was recommended. A dilation and curettage (D & C) indicated that Linda had suffered a hydatidiform molar pregnancy, a rare condition in which the decaying placental tissues burrow into the uterine wall and begin to grow. Left unchecked, these tissues can degenerate into a fast-growing cancer.

A second D & C was performed in January 1980. During the procedure the physician unintentionally removed too much of Linda's uterine lining, making it difficult for a fertilized egg to adhere to the surface. But the bad news didn't end there. The tumor, which the physician thought was benign, had begun to grow again. Calling the McRobbies into his office, the gynecologist told them the tumor was cancerous. He wanted to begin treatment as soon as possible. Linda was so distraught that she couldn't even walk to the car. Glenn finally picked her up and carried her. She sobbed most of the long drive home. If there ever was a black day in the McRobbies' lives, they say this was the blackest.

In the years since, Linda has done her best to tune out this chapter of her life. But try as she might, she hasn't managed to erase the memory of that day when she learned she had cancer. "At my age finding out that you are pregnant and a whole new life is growing in you . . . well, I was overwhelmed with happiness," she said, looking back. "Then to learn I had cancer . . . I was crushed. I panicked. I didn't think I would survive. This beautiful baby had turned into a horrible monster of cells gone crazy." Even worse was her innate knowledge that she would never bear children. No one had told Linda this. She wasn't even fully aware of how seriously the gynecologist had damaged her uterine lining. She just sensed instinctively that she was infertile.

With her marriage to Glenn Linda had managed to bury her premonition of infertility. Infused with her husband's zest for life, she often forgot her trepidation. In Glenn's eyes anything was possible if you tried hard enough. And Linda tried hard, but what worked for him didn't always work for her. Sometimes she resented his single-minded pursuit of children. But the annoyance was always transitory. When she became sick Glenn remained her main source of solace, comfort, and support. He was always there for her, no matter how tough or discouraging the situation became.

On February 14, 1980 a large brick hospital became Linda's home. There she lived for four months, receiving chemotherapy treatment each day for five days in a row. The doctors gave her a week off, then resumed treatment. Between February and September she received at least fifty chemotherapy shots, each one as debilitating as the last.

During this time Linda lived in constant dread that the medicine wouldn't be effective. She was in a cancer ward. She witnessed deaths. She even heard that a baby had died of the disease. Every day she lived with the reality of her own mortality. After three weeks in the hospital she felt as if she was going crazy. She found it impossible to sleep, and without sleep she soon became a physical and an emotional wreck. The only blessing in all this misery was that she had little energy left for dwelling on her miscarriage or her child-bearing prospects. She felt fortunate that she had lost the fetus too soon to become attached to or fantasize about it. While she was hospitalized she had no thoughts of children. "Mostly, I worried about other people's reactions to me. People act funny when you have cancer," she reflected.

As winter slowly turned to spring, Linda's health began to improve. Still, there was no guarantee of complete recovery. The doctors warned the McRobbies that there was always the possiblity Linda might develop an immunity to the medicine. For Glenn this was a constant worry. By April, with her blood count close to normal, Linda teetered between the hope of complete recovery and the fear that the cancer would reemerge to consume her. Allowed to return home every other week during this harrowing period, she remembers sitting on a rock at the back of her home and crying simply because she could smell the air.

Believing Linda to be cured, the doctors sent her home at the end of the month. Her relief was intense. Both McRobbies were physically and emotionally drained. Linda, however, was still experiencing physical problems. When her period was due she suffered excruciating pain, but there was no menstruation. Despite this nagging concern her blood tests returned to normal in May and June, and she was able to resume most of her activities. She and Glenn even took the time to explore the possibility of adopting a child and registered with both a Catholic and a secular adoption agency near their home. But before they could get caught up in the adoption process, they were overwhelmed by the news that Linda's cancer had returned and was growing again. She was told that she would have to repeat the entire surgical and chemical procedure.

Hearing the news, Linda broke down and wept in the doctor's office. By the next week, though, she had rallied and was submitting to yet another D & C. It revealed little cancerous material, and the physician believed that whatever remained could be knocked out with chemotherapy. The bad news was that Linda's chances of bearing children had diminished even more. Although she would probably be able to menstruate, her doctor said he doubted that she would ever be able to carry a child.

The end of Linda's cancer ordeal came on September 13, 1980, the date of her last chemotherapy treatment. But the long emotional rehabilitation process was still ahead. It would be two years before Linda regained confidence in her health. "For a year," she said, "I would shake whenever I took a blood test." Then there was the worry over whether she would ever menstruate again. She and Glenn were well aware that a natural pregnancy—even the use of eggs for in vitro fertilization or embryo transplant—was impossible without menstruation. Then, irony of ironies, as soon as Linda was off chemotherapy, her gynecologist put her on the birth control pill. Besides preventing her from becoming pregnant—not likely, but still possible—the pill was supposed to clear up the question of whether the cancer had regenerated. The hormones released during pregnancy are the same as those released by cancerous tumors of the kind that afflicted Linda. Without the pill, there was no way of knowing whether she was pregnant or the tumor had returned.

For the McRobbies the pill was an annoyance, a real and symbolic barrier to pregnancy. When almost a year had passed, Linda took herself off the pill and began to use other forms of birth control. She was anxious to find out whether she could get her period without artificial means. Within a month, she was menstruating for the first time in almost two years. Her time of darkness was over, or so she thought.

Now that it was possible to resume attempts at conception, Linda found that she no longer had a great deal of enthusiasm for the process. She was physically repulsed by the thought of giving birth. Deep down, but unspoken for fear of hurting Glenn, she felt a compelling desire to say no to pregnancy. In fact, she secretly prayed that an adoption agency would provide them with a child. She felt she needed time to heal. Glenn had only an inkling of her true feelings. For almost two years he had stood on the sidelines while his wife faced death. He couldn't help feeling he had waited long enough. It was time to see if they could have children.

Linda acceded to her husband's wishes for a variety of reasons. Her knowledge of his previous marriage and divorce made her afraid of losing him if she refused to have children. She also had a deep-seated need to provide her parents with a grandchild. So with these thoughts to spur her on, but less than enthusiastically, she went along with the pregnancy attempts. Her only condition was that they work on natural pregnancy and adoption simultaneously.

Glenn soon dubbed this period—which lasted for three years—"the pits." Until this point in their marriage he had been relegated to the role of handholder and chief negotiator with the myriad of physicians who had come in and out of their lives. Now, it seemed, it was his turn to suffer. For the first time in his life Glenn found himself in the uncomfortable position of having to perform on demand. During Linda's menstrual cycle he was fine for the most part. But when ovulation time rolled around he was almost paralyzed by his fear of being impotent. For a while he actually toyed with the idea of being hypnotized or even freezing his sperm for later use. He liked the idea of whipping out a vial and handing the worry over to someone else.

On several occasions during these years Linda believed

that she was pregnant and had miscarried. Both she and Glenn became more despondent as the months passed without a viable pregnancy. Glenn decided to set a timetable for continuing with their attempts at a natural pregnancy; they would give themselves ten years. If Linda hadn't conceived by the time he was forty-five, he was determined to explore alternate reproductive technologies. The situation was doubly hard on Linda. She was the one who had undergone the physical agony of at least one miscarriage, and perhaps more, of several D & C's, and cancer treatment. She still found routine gynecological exams emotionally and physically draining. Now, for the sake of a dream, she had to submit to one painful fertility test after another.

The worst of these was the hysterogram, a specialized X-ray that determines whether the fallopian tubes are clear. Linda recalls lying on a narrow examining table while her doctor inserted the X-ray instrument into her cervix. All her pelvic muscles contracted, and she heard her screams fill the small room. Finally, after what seemed an eternity, the instrument was removed. "I bled for five days from that thing," Linda said, still angry many years later at the test and the manner in which it was administered on that one occasion. "I'm sure it was worse than giving birth," she decided. And for a long while afterward her nightmares returned—nightmares of the cancer ward and death.

Although she tried not to dwell on the question of her fertility, Linda agonized a great deal in private over whether to put a halt to the pregnancy attempts. Sometimes, when she was particularly despondent, she would tell herself that she was infertile and the whole process was a waste of time. But when her period was late, hope was rekindled. She would begin counting the days only to face disappointment once again. If only things could be one way or another, she told herself. If only she could find a way off this treadmill without hurting Glenn and their marriage.

Weeks passed, then months and years. The more Glenn

pushed for Linda to continue this sisyphean routine, the more she resented him. At times the resentment was so great that she wasn't sure she would be able to stay with him. "His intensity scared me," she later admitted. "I thought it was consuming him. I felt he was out of whack and we were out of whack. At one point I thought it would be best to free him of the marriage; there was such a hole there. I wondered if I might not cause him more misery by staying. I felt very much alone. Then I'd look at our family tree and realize that it was going to end with me. I'd think, 'I'll never be able to give my parents a grandchild.' "

Fueled in part by an intense need to show the world she was whole, Linda persevered. She wanted to show all the doctors she had visited that they were mistaken about her infertility. For her, having a child was a symbol of health. And despite her annoyance with Glenn, Linda counted on him to keep her going. When she found herself in a funk or fit of depression, wondering whether the pain and upset would ever end, Glenn was there to comfort her. He was there for her, as well, when her father died in December of 1983. This was not only one of the most difficult moments of Linda's life but a major turning point in her attitude toward fertility.

The onset of what turned out to be very advanced pancreatic cancer had actually started the summer before with flu-like symptoms. And by October, after massive weight loss, Linda's father had to be hospitalized. The doctors at the veterans hospital gave him two months to live. The burden of the elderly man's care fell mainly on Linda, who, apart from Glenn, had to deal with the terror and pain of her father's sickness virtually alone. Together they visited him every other day in his drab hospital room. And even though he was visibly suffering from the chemotherapy, Linda would lie and tell him that he was getting better. After about a month of hospitalization, he begged to be allowed to leave and was brought home for his birthday on November 16.

Linda says she will never forget the cribbage game she had with her father on the afternoon of his birthday. He was so sick and depressed that he could barely concentrate on the board. She felt there had to be some way to cheer him up. Remembering that her period was late, she told her father she thought she was pregnant. Hearing the happy news the sick man sat up, looking a hundred times better. "I sure hope it's true," he said, patting Linda on the knee. He died the following month still believing that she would bear him a grandchild, mentioning it just before his death on a rainy Tuesday evening in December. Delayed by the weather Glenn and Linda had arrived at the hospital later than usual. Linda's father had died half an hour earlier, sitting up in bed with his hair combed and his mustache trimmed, awaiting their arrival.

For six months following her father's death Linda had trouble sleeping. For a while she even stopped ovulating. As she emerged from her mourning period she said an emphatic no to additional fertility testing and only halfheartedly agreed to attempt to get pregnant without drugs. She told herself that she was sick of "all that fertility stuff" and had to give up what she now felt was the futile hope of getting pregnant. But, for all that, she was no less intent on having a family. "A life is taken, a life is given." The words echoed in her mind throughout the long, dreary winter months after the death. The dream of presenting her father with a grandchild—even posthumously—was very much alive. Now, however, Linda decided they would depend on adoption or some alternate means of producing the family unit she and Glenn so yearned for.

The McRobbies had taken their first, tentative steps toward adoption in the spring of 1980 when Linda was released from the netherworld of the cancer ward. Both she and Glenn were optimistic about their chances of being accepted. After all, they were hardworking professionals who could well afford to provide a child with a comfortable home. One evening in mid-July of that year the McRobbies, along with about ten other nervous couples, gathered in the austere, institutional conference room of the headquarters of a Catholic adoption agency near their home. Glenn remembers observing that there were people from all different socioeconomic brackets at the meeting. "Everyone was a little nervous and shy," he said, looking back. "And everyone wanted a baby yesterday." Linda, in turn, saw "a room filled with devastating emotions, with wide-eyed people full of a sense of false hope. We all wanted the woman to say, 'We're going to give you all kids, don't worry,' "

The bland, middle-aged woman who entered the room said no such thing. In fact, she couldn't have been more discouraging. An agency supervisor, she advised the couples in the room that their wait for a child would be long and arduous. The supply of babies was dwindling, it seemed. It could be several years before the agency started a home study, and several more before parents accepted for adoption could hope to receive a child. Glenn took an immediate dislike to the woman. Instead of finding the warm, sympathetic person he had expected, he felt he was in the presence of a disapproving school marm. He was sick at heart at being forced to approach people he didn't like for something as special as a child. As a Protestant, he also felt distinctly out of place in a Catholic environment.

About a week after attending the introductory meeting at the Catholic agency, the McRobbies attended another meeting at a secular adoption agency. Glenn found its employees patronizing, and the McRobbies didn't have to wait long before they were told that this agency couldn't help them either. The negative messages emanating from both adoption agencies made the McRobbies feel more desperate than they had before embarking on this course. At least before, despite the cancer, there had been some hope of adopting a child. Now that route, too, seemed virtually closed to them. However they had little choice but to continue.

What the McRobbies came to know firsthand from these experiences was the sad but true picture of domestic adoption in the 1980s. Changes in abortion laws, more effective birth control, and a trend toward single mothers raising their own children had combined to shrink the available pool of healthy babies to such an extent that by 1987 it was possible for a couple to wait as much as eight years to adopt an American-born child in some parts of the country. Their experience with these agencies had already convinced the McRobbies that adoption of a healthy white child would be no picnic, a view shared by many infertile couples.

Writing about her own adoption experience for the Association Press, Janet Staihar described domestic adoption as "a maze of wrong turns, doubts and sheer luck." In the course of research on the subject and personal involvement with the process, she encountered couples "so frustrated with the red tape and requirements of adopting babies domestically that some [resorted to paying] bogus adoption services for Mexican babies who perhaps never existed." Other couples have been so put off by the formal adoption process that they have attempted to work out adoptions directly with a willing biological mother. And there are those who, like the McRobbies, have turned to surrogate parenting as a means of alleviating the particular brand of heartbreak that seems to be meted out by the adoption agencies. But they didn't turn to surrogacy immediately. For despite those first, depressing encounters with adoption agencies, in the spring of 1980 neither Glenn nor Linda was prepared to forgo adoption as a possibility.

Linda was neither physically nor emotionally prepared to venture into the realm of the new reproductive technologies such as surrogate parenting. And Glenn simply went along with adoption to please her but was never able to muster any enthusiasm for the process. From the beginning he hated the lack of control the process offered infertile couples, the waiting, and the ultimate indignity of having to rely totally on strangers for something as precious as a baby. And like most husbands of infertile women, he really wanted his own child.

Glenn had learned about surrogate parenting from a television show he had seen that winter and was prepared to go that route immediately. Out of consideration for Linda and her recent cancer experience, however, he delayed broaching the topic. He sensed that she wasn't ready to relinquish her natural role as the mother of his child to another woman. However neither of the McRobbies was prepared for the four-year battle that followed—a devastating battle filled with untold ups and downs, with an emotionally damaging examination of their religious beliefs, and ultimately, with disappointment.

On the advice of their minister they decided to focus their efforts on the Catholic agency because it was the largest in the area and offered the greatest supply of babies. The first of many jolts from that source came several weeks after the McRobbies attended the agency's introductory session. That was when they received a letter from the agency questioning the status of their marriage. Unbelievable as it then seemed, the agency did not consider the McRobbies legally married in the eyes of the Roman Catholic church. They had both previously been married to and divorced from Catholics and there was no record of an annulment in either case.

As distraught as the McRobbies were about this news, they were made more so by the discovery that Linda's cancer had returned at the end of July. For the time being, the McRobbies had to put adoption on the back burner. Then, in December, they received another letter regarding their marriage. The agency now informed them that unless they could secure annulments, adoption through their office would be out of the question. Angry beyond words the McRobbies nevertheless opted to stay with the Catholic agency. Their minister had managed a successful adoption of his own thanks to these people and he urged them to stick it out, even if it meant obtaining annulments. So, at his insistence, both Linda and Glenn swallowed their anger and pride and began to prepare material for the Catholic marriage tribunal.

Linda, who had been brought up in the Catholic faith and later converted to Protestantism, found the annulment process far more traumatic than Glenn did. For him the procedure was "just another pain in the ass," one more step along the long route to getting a child. Once the annulments were complete and the slates were clean, he thought their candidacy for adoption would be secure. Linda simply hated the whole awful business and barely pushed herself along in the hope of getting a child.

The annulment hearings were scheduled for May 1981. Both Glenn and Linda returned to the agency for separate interviews and were granted annulments by August. With this out of the way the agency kept its word and put the McRobbies on their home-study list, making them eligible for consideration if they were found to be suitable. They now learned what most adopting couples in the 1980s take for granted: adoption is a lengthy process. It would be three years—until September 1984—before this particular agency got to their case. Throughout this three-year period the McRobbies had actively pursued other adoption possibilities and by April 1984 they were prepared to move in one of three directions. They were at the top of the list at a small secular agency—one with a smaller pool of babies than its Catholic counterpart—were close to being scheduled for a home study at the Catholic agency, and had the opportunity to adopt a Polish émigré baby.

The McRobbies had friends who had adopted a Polish emigre baby, and reminded of her own Polish background, Linda thought this would be a wonderful way of honoring her father. These same friends put the McRobbies in touch with Polish officials in New York. The main drawbacks were the price—what then seemed a prohibitive $12,000—

and the political unrest taking place in Poland at the time. There was no guarantee they would be able to get a child out of the country. After a good deal of discussion, including another talk with their minister, the McRobbies opted to have their name dropped from the list at the secular agency rather than jeopardize their chances at the larger Catholic agency. Although it is possible to maintain multiple applications at a variety of adoption agencies, most establishments require that their applicants work solely with them once the home-study process has begun.

Finally, on a sunny day in June, Glenn and Linda were rewarded for their patience. Almost four years to the day on which they had originally applied to the Catholic agency for adoption, they received notice that a preliminary home-study meeting was scheduled for July. At this session the McRobbies filled out more applications, produced references, and paid a $100 fee. They would be assigned a social worker when the results of the mandatory physicals had been processed. There was only one hitch. The supervisor conducting the session informed them that the annulments hadn't cleared up the question of Linda's religious status. A priest who specialized in canon law was studying the matter.

The McRobbies left the supervisor's office feeling slightly dismayed. What did this new development mean? In the absence of any answers, they forged ahead with the necessary physicals. Half of the summer passed with no word from the agency. Unable to wait any longer, Glenn called the office on August 1 and learned that staff vacations had delayed the start of their home-study. A social worker had been assigned to their case, however, and planned to contact them in September.

The home-study section of the adoption procedure consisted of seven meetings with a social worker, stretching from September to November of 1984. From the beginning the McRobbies were displeased with the social worker who was sent to judge them and their life-style. They soon realized that she would not be the comforting, motherly figure of their fantasies. She was businesslike, slightly officious, and no help at all when it came to clarifying the agency's concern over religious issues. Still, she was their only hope. They made every effort to be open with this woman and to comply with her wishes. When she asked Linda to write a statement of faith, Linda did so even though she found the task repugnant. Things seemed to be proceeding so well that she hated to do anything that might derail the adoption. And everything they had been hearing from the social worker was optimistic. The beautiful fall weather they had been having seemed a sign of good things to come, and they exulted—and hoped.

But even as the warmest fall day brings a hint of winter, so even the social worker's most encouraging comments began to be tinged with one warning or another. On more than one occasion she assured the McRobbies that she would recommend them for adoption as long as the church was satisfied with Linda's religious status. But she saved the worst for their final session, which took place in the McRobbies' home one cold November afternoon. After a tour of the house, which she noted was extremely clean, the woman ensconced herself on the living room couch and proceeded to fire away with a barrage of questions and criticisms. She found Glenn too cold and reserved and worried that he never expressed anger. As for Linda, she was informed that she had committed "informal heresy" by leaving the church. Linda's conversion to Protestantism was a problem. How bad a problem, though, she couldn't say.

After listening to the McRobbies' protests, the woman stowed her notebook in her bag and prepared to leave. Once again she was the pleasant, if stern, social worker who had seemed so encouraging at their other sessions. Once again she assured them that she would give them her wholehearted recommendation. And once again she made no promise that Linda's conversion would not prove a stumbling block to their acceptance as adoptive parents. When they closed the door behind her the McRobbies could feel nothing but dismay. Linda, who was emotionally drained and exhausted from the ordeal, now thought of the woman as her enemy. She said she didn't believe her parting words of encouragement and was sure the adoption would never happen.

Linda was right about the adoption. One clear, cold afternoon in December the McRobbies were summoned to the agency for official notification that their adoption application had been denied. Seated on hard wooden chairs grouped around a table were the adoption supervisor and the social worker who had handled their case. Linda's conversion to the Protestant faith was given as the cause. There was also a secondary concern—one that had not come up during the long home-study process. The adoption committee feared that Linda's illness and her father's recent death were emotional handicaps. They questioned her ability to cope with an energetic child.

At first the McRobbies were too outraged to respond. Struggling for composure, Glenn finally argued that the tragedies Linda had faced made her an excellent candidate for motherhood. But the agency, it seemed, had built an airtight case for denial. Every time Glenn countered one of their criticisms, one of the two women came up with another to take its place. They were concerned, for example, with whether the McRobbies would be willing to wait two more years—the time it might take to find a Protestant baby. Unable to stand it any longer, Linda ran out of the room sobbing. Glenn found her crying in the car when the meeting broke up about half an hour later. She told him she wanted to get as far from them as possible. But first she wanted to shake them and say, "I'm a good person. Can't you see?" It seemed that all those meetings had been nothing but a circle of confusion and contradiction. She wanted to tell them that Jesus wouldn't have judged her the way they had. That night the McRobbies debated whether to appeal the agency's decision. Glenn felt they should, but he made one stipulation. He had contacted a surrogate parenting center in a nearby city several weeks earlier and wanted to go through with the appointment. To his surprise Linda had no objections. He fell asleep that night feeling confident that they would have a child.

Glenn had finally made the decision to push for surrogate parenting in October, while driving around on business calls. At that point they had been immersed in the home-study and he was sick of the whole adoption process. "I'd had enough," he said. "I'd been on the outside looking in. I had no fertility problems, no religious problems."

And, as was his habit when making important decisions, he made a pact with himself to wait a month before acting. If he still felt as strongly about surrogacy following the home-study, he would discuss it with Linda. As it turned out, Linda was so disgusted with the adoption decision that she was willing to try just about anything.

The adoption appeal was scheduled for late December. Protest as Glenn might, the agency officials would not budge from their position. Denial was upheld. The McRobbies left the room convinced that the religious question had played a major role in the agency's decision. That night Glenn began to prepare notes for a lawsuit. By the time he had released all his anger on paper—twenty-five pages worth—he no longer had the desire to sue. Moreover, he and Linda no longer had the money. They were building a house and planning to spend at least $20,000 to have a child—$10,000 to be paid to the surrogate parenting clinic, and $10,000 to be held in escrow for the woman who would bear their child.

# 3 | A Dream Realized: The Surrogate Parenting Process

Just before Christmas 1984 Glenn and Linda received the most precious of gifts—the gift of renewed hope. It was on that day that Elaine Silver, a psychiatric social worker and the director of a nearby surrogate parenting clinic, accepted the McRobbies into her program as prospective parents. Suddenly a whole, magical world of family and children opened to them. The dream, which had sustained them through the fertility tests, the cancer, and the adoption attempts, was achievable. Perhaps they wouldn't be parents that day, the next, or even in nine months, but the possibility now existed. Moreover, in Elaine the McRobbies found the empathetic soul they had longed for throughout their adoption experience. As an infertile woman, Elaine knew firsthand the sufferings of infertile couples. And she knew firsthand the joy of easing that pain by matching those couples with someone who would bear their child. By that December she had seven successful births to her record.

After years of rejection, years of people telling them they

didn't measure up physically, emotionally, or even spiritually, it was with some trepidation that Glenn and Linda set out that blustery winter afternoon for their appointment at the surrogate parenting clinic. Nervous, depressed, terrified of being judged again, they were making the trek out of sheer desperation. They felt that this was their last resort. Not surprisingly, neither Glenn nor Linda talked much during the hour-long ride. Even Glenn was depressed and fast losing hope. He figured this was "the last inning."

The McRobbies had no trouble finding the bustling community in which the clinic was located, and the large, austere medical building Elaine had described soon became visible. But it was some time before they found the clinic, which was marked only by a small metal sign attached to the door. A pleasant-looking woman in her mid-thirties, Elaine answered their tentative knock with a friendly greeting. Leading them into a small office decorated in soothing shades, the director of the clinic suggested that they take a seat on a soft, ivory-colored sofa. Before long, Linda found she had stopped shaking and her hands no longer were sweating. She had been waiting for Elaine to bombard them with questions. Instead, this woman seemed genuinely sympathetic to their plight. "I ended up spilling out my story and my feelings," she recalled. And, to Linda's surprise and relief no judgment was passed. For his part Glenn was relieved to note Elaine's indifference to religion. "All she cared about was whether we wanted kids—whether we both wanted them," he said, looking back. If they had had mixed feelings about having kids, it seems, she would have sent them packing.

With all the ease the McRobbies felt with Elaine, they never forgot that she represented what they believed to be their last hope of having a child. For that reason, they held back something of themselves. There was the fear that revealing too much—about Linda's medical history, for example, or the rejection by the Catholic agency—would once again trigger that most painful of words "no." Certainly they never expected to hear "yes" that day. But halfway through the appointment Elaine announced that she would accept them into her program. "Let's get going," she told the McRobbies, transforming them at one fell swoop from an infertile couple with almost no hope of having a child into prospective parents.

Both Linda and Glenn were too stunned and elated to react, let alone question the speed of Elaine's decision. A whole new world was beckoning. That house they were building would need a nursery and a basketball court. They were going to have a baby. Amazing. They didn't stop to consider Elaine's casual style; it seemed appropriate to them. They were too elated to give any thought to such details as screening or background checks. They were too excited to pause and think that Elaine was making a major commitment to them based solely on her own assessment of them. What they instinctively concluded was that Elaine was a great judge of character. Glenn, for one, didn't need to ask many questions. He knew that surrogate parenting involved risks—and he was prepared to take them. If the state of Massachusetts—like most states in the country—didn't recognize surrogate parenting, so be it. If a court of law didn't uphold their contract, so be it. If a surrogate reneged and insisted on keeping the baby, they would fight her in court. They would simply cross those bridges when they got there.

The risks inherent in surrogate parenting—the possibility of confused paternity, surrogates who balked, legal tangles—frightened Linda much more than they did Glenn. But Elaine's optimism was contagious. The McRobbies soon realized that the opportunity to have someone else bear a child for them was too wonderful to sacrifice to such worries. "We had to do it," Linda later said.

"There were no 'ifs', 'ands', or 'buts' about it. You do it and live with the fear." She found reassurance in what was then the clinic's policy of retaining strict anonymity between surrogate mothers and couples. For her, it was tremendously important that this remain a business transaction—no more or less. The thought of becoming personally involved with the surrogate was too threatening. It was enough to know the woman's first name and the state in which she lived.

On the way home Linda confessed that she was worried about the $20,000 they would have to spend for a child. She was also afraid of the surrogate's power over the baby. Glenn, who couldn't wait to get going, did his best to dilute her anxieties. What was the money, he argued, when this was their last chance to be parents? How could they put a price tag on a child? By the time they arrived home, he had her convinced that the $20,000 was a trifling amount.

That night the McRobbies sat down at their kitchen table and pored over the multipage contract Elaine had given them to review with their lawyer. So many words, so many conditions. The longer Linda and Glenn studied the contract, the more convinced they became that all would be well. Whatever the risks Elaine had outlined in her office, they now paled before the McRobbies' mutual fantasy of a smiling, gurgling baby to love and cherish. For Linda this would be the fulfillment of the promise she had made to her father before he died. For Glenn it was the fulfillment of a lifetime dream.

But in the days that followed, days filled with lawyers and contract signings, one gnawing fear returned again and again to haunt Linda. What would happen if the surrogate refused to relinquish the baby? Her spirits were so buoyant, however, that she felt this was no more than a speck of dust against an otherwise crystalline sky. Yet in quiet, still moments when Glenn wasn't around to boost her morale, the worry resurfaced, causing little ripples in her peace. But things evolved so rapidly that Linda had no time to dwell on her fears.

Two days after Christmas the McRobbies were back at the surrogate parenting clinic—this time to select the woman they hoped would bear their child. Sifting through Elaine's files, they came across a Denver, Colorado woman named Alice who seemed to personify the wholesomeness they were seeking. There was only one hitch. Alice was planning to move to a southern state within the month. If she accepted them as a suitable couple, they would have to postpone insemination until the move was completed. Glenn and Linda breathed a collective sigh.

Now that they had found a woman to bear their child, the McRobbies wanted to get her pregnant as soon as possible. But Glenn's gung-ho spirit was jolted by the gory details of artificial insemination. For the required sperm test he would have to masturbate into a cup. Worst of all was the fact that Linda wasn't allowed to help. Elaine was adamant about that—no withdrawal techniques. She insisted that the best sperm, the first to be ejaculated, might be lost. "Everyone gets nervous," she assured him. "When you get nervous, think baby and everything will be fine."

As it turned out, Linda was able to play at least a bit part in the insemination process. While arranging the dreaded sperm test, Glenn learned that she could assist in arousing him without damaging "the product." Once the masturbation issue was resolved, though, he began to fret about his performance. With the mention of artificial insemination all sexual desire had gone. What if he was impotent? he asked Linda several days before the sperm test was scheduled. What if he failed? She suggested he stock up on "girlie" magazines and even proposed that they make the purchase a family outing. The night before the test the two of them ventured out to a newsstand that carried pornography. Unfortunately, the store was smack in the center of the financial district in which Glenn worked. Linda panicked about meeting someone they knew. Her idea of decorous conduct under the circumstances was to grab a few magazines, pay for them as quickly as possible, and stash them in the brief-case Glenn was carrying. In the end a red-faced Linda had to drag her husband out of the store. At home they spent the the evening chortling over Glenn's purchaes.

Glenn was scheduled to appear at a local hospital with his jar of sperm by 8:00 A.M. on Monday. Looking back, he said, "I sweated bullets all weekend reading those dumb magazines. I read so many of them that by Sunday night when I was lying in bed all I could see were bodies in all sorts of positions. I reached over and nudged Linda and told her, 'I think I'm overprepared. I may have a wet dream.' " That night Glenn was so terrified of impotency that he couldn't sleep. When the alarm went off at 7:15, Linda laughingly jostled him. He reached for the jar on his bedstand and wondered again whether he would be able to do it. The whole process took about thirty seconds. After showering and dressing in a rush to make his appointment, Glenn ran out of the house with the jar under his arm, a precaution necessary to keep the sperm warm. He drove to the hospital and wandered around the large building in search of the right laboratory. All the while he was terrified that the sperm would die and he would have to repeat the entire, humiliating procedure.

Four hours later the doctor called and said, "Well, super-man, your sperm count is above average and the sperm are extremely active." Exhilarated by the report, Glenn called Linda. Knowing her hyperactive husband, she wasn't particularly surprised by this report. But try as she might, she couldn't help gloating over Glenn's insemination ordeal. "For once," she explained, "he had all the pressure." Moreover, with the spotlight on him, Linda found she could really relax for the first time in five years. "It was such a great relief to have another woman take over," she later admitted, "I didn't feel any jealousy. I was only thrilled that we were getting a chance to have a baby and this other woman was taking the burden off my shoulders."

The first week in January Elaine phoned with the happy news that Alice had accepted the McRobbies. The bad news was that Elaine suggested they postpone the insemination until after Alice's move. They agreed. But one month merged into three. In April Alice was still wavering between a boyfriend in one state and a job in another. At this point Glenn and Linda decided to find another surrogate. With Alice out of the picture, though, Glenn became restless. Elaine had been screening a few women as potential surrogates, but there was no immediate replacement. Unless they started shopping around for a surrogate mother on their own, they were stuck for the present. But neither of the McRobbies particularly wanted to be involved in the screening process. Linda, especially, wanted emotional distance from the woman who would bear their child because she felt this would lessen the chances that the surrogate would want to keep the baby.

Before desperation could set in, Elaine called with information on another prospective surrogate. The woman's name was Helen, and she was the single mother of a little girl. Elaine was particularly excited about Helen because she appeared to be similar to Linda in coloring, height, and weight. Moreover, she had tall brothers, which pleased Glenn because he didn't want to produce a "midget." There were other positive things about Helen that pleased the McRobbies. She came from an intact nuclear family, had a good health profile, and didn't seem to be in surrogate parenting just for the money, which would have disqualified her from Elaine's program automatically. She also lived relatively close by, within driving distance, which would cut down on the cost and time involved in traveling for the inseminations. Because only fresh semen was used in Elaine's surrogate parenting clinic, Glenn had to appear in person for each attempt.

By now Linda realized that the surrogate had to satisfy four basic requirements: she had to be psychologically stable; have decent physical characteristics; good health, and values that were similar to theirs. The fact that Helen resembled Linda was an added inducement to selecting her. The McRobbies were further sold on her clean medical and psychological record. When Elaine called back later that day to announce that Helen had agreed to bear their child, Linda felt that fate had thrown them together. To Glenn this meant they were back on track and he could feel good again.

Thus began one of the most peculiar relationships anyone could have devised. Overnight, the surrogate's menstrual cycle, health, appearance, and life-style became of the greatest importance to the McRobbies. Yet Helen was more mirage than person to them. They had never seen or talked with her, and they knew very little about her beyond the sketchy material Elaine had provided. And yet, sight unseen, the three of them had contracted to be involved in one of the most intimate of human activities—the creation of a life. If the McRobbies seemed caught up in the mechanics of making this arrangement work—ovulation, artificial insemination, conception—the magnitude of their pact with Helen was never lost on them. Linda found herself constantly thinking about the woman—imagining her appearance, how she spent her day. She also read and reread Helen's profile until she became "a part of my life." Nonetheless, in reality the McRobbies' relationship with Helen remained on of fantasy while their bond remained technical, which was precisely how they wanted it. If they allowed Helen to get too close, they feared they might not be able to let her go. And she in turn might not let the baby go.

The first test of the viability of the surrogacy arrangement came in mid-May when Elaine informed the McRobbies that Helen would be ovulating at the end of the month. They had to be prepared to get to the clinic as soon as they received word that Helen was fertile. About a week later, Linda called Glenn at his office to tell him that Helen was indeed ovulating. Glenn's big moment had arrived. He stopped to pick up Linda and they headed out to the clinic. Throughout the drive Glenn was so preoccupied with what he regarded as his impending fate that by the time they had pulled into the parking lot, he was just going through the motions. In retrospect he said, "I walked into the building with Linda and I knew that half an hour from now I would either have a smile on my face or be the most depressed guy in America. I figured I would be the only one to fail. I didn't care if anyone laughed, but I didn't want to fail."

As they started down the long corridor leading to the wing that housed Elaine's clinic, Glenn could hear his steps echoing. The sound filled him with an uncontrollable feeling of fear and trembling. He was relieved when Elaine's husband answered their knock. Today of all days, he wanted no lectures on "thinking baby." Explaining that his wife had been called out on an emergency, Elaine's husband handed Glenn a sample jar, instructed him on its use, and gave him the number of the doctor's office to call when he was finished. Helen would be upstairs awaiting the sample.

As the main office door closed behind them, the McRobbies proceeded to undress in a small sitting room. As he removed article after article of clothing, Glenn felt his life pass before him. When he was completely naked, he glanced down and was dismayed at the sight of his inert penis. "My God, Linda," he mumbled, "It's receding." She grinned and continued to undress. Standing naked in the sitting room of a strange professional office, Glenn's only thought was of getting it over with. The main problem was that the couch was too small to accommodate his tall frame. The most comfortable place was the floor. Totally consumed with laughter, Linda joined Glenn on the carpet.

"It's come to this," he said to her as she nestled beside him. "Lying on an office floor trying to have a kid. If anyone had told me ten years ago that this was what I would need to do to have a family, I would have said they were out of their minds." He had one moment of panic when he couldn't locate the jar, but otherwise everything went smoothly. Ten minutes later the McRobbies were back in their car, having dressed quickly and carried the sample to the doctor's office upstairs. That was it. Now all they could do was wait.

As they pulled out of the parking lot Linda found herself chuckling at the thought of the two of them on a stranger's floor. She was glad she had given in to Glenn's urgings to help out. She felt this made her a part of the baby's creation. The following days were a harrowing vigil of wait and see. Concentrating on the day-to-day routine with a major drama unfolding two hundred miles away was unbelievably difficult. When they calculated that Helen's period was late they went "right off the walls" every time the phone rang. After a week without news, Glenn called the clinic. Elaine confirmed that Helen's period was indeed late but said she didn't expect any additional information for another week.

Although they were ecstatic at the news, the McRobbies didn't bring out the champagne or schedule a celebration. They reminded each other that it was stupid to get excited; inflated expectations too often led to unbearable disappointment. But after all those dreary years, they couldn't restrain themselves from conjuring up one sweet image after another of baby and family and home. When Helen's delayed period turned out to be a false alarm, their disappointment was intense. To Glenn it was as if someone had played a cruel joke on them. Linda went up to their bedroom and cried. That night Glenn lay awake for hours wondering why they couldn't have been spared this particular letdown.

The next day both of the McRobbies realized that they had been overly optimistic. After all, this was only the first month, the first attempt at insemination. "We should have controlled our emotions," Linda said later, "but we couldn't help it." What helped them bounce back was the realization that Helen's next ovulation was only two weeks away. The only problem was that she was expected to be most fertile right in the middle of the long July Fourth weekend when the clinic would be closed. Elaine suggested that the McRobbies try later in the week, even though there was no guarantee that Helen would still be fertile.

Why not, they decided, arranging to leave work early on July 8. Linda's mother lived a short distance from the clinic, and they drove over there to produce the sperm sample, knowing she was away for the week. Glenn was a little uncomfortable but decided that sex in his mother-in-law's house was preferable to the clinic floor. With the sperm jar lodged firmly under Linda's armpit to ensure warmth, they raced to the doctor's office where Helen was waiting. Making the drop-off, Linda felt like a fool as she wandered strange corridors with the jar under her arm. When she finally located the right office, she thrust the sperm sample on the receptionist's desk and ran out without giving her name. For a few days she fretted that her hasty actions might have caused a mix-up. But when no one had called after a week, the McRobbies once again took up the obsessive calendar watch. This time they were more cautious, more detached. Helen's period was late again, but they refused to call the clinic. However, they could only hold off for so long. After another week of unbearable waiting, Glenn called and learned that Helen had gone for a blood test. The results had been lost, and she had gone for another test. Elaine promised to get back to them as soon as she had any news.

Four or five days passed without a word from Elaine. Glenn was just about to leave work for the day that Friday when he got a call from her. "Congratulations," she said in a pleased voice. "You're going to be a father." He was totally taken aback. For years he had been waiting to hear those words. Now that he had, he was catatonic. Overhearing the conversation his secretary relayed the news to the rest of the office. Soon there were a half-dozen people hovering around Glenn cheering and clapping. Elaine found Linda at home. "I was dumbfounded and ecstatic," she said. "When I finally heard the word pregnant, I couldn't believe it."

That night, in a fog of emotion, the McRobbies went to a Chinese restaurant to celebrate. The only thing that mattered was that they had each other and would soon have the baby. How they got to the restaurant and how they got home again is still a mystery to them.

During those early days of the pregnancy there was little concern about Helen and what she might do with the baby. The McRobbies' only thought was for her health and progress. Linda found herself constantly praying that everything would be all right—that the labor would be short and the baby wouldn't be deformed. She was only an "onlooker." But at this stage she was a contented onlooker. Glenn stayed up in the clouds for a week after learning that he would be a father. When he drove the car he found himself honking his horn and waving happily to people. "I was elated," he said. "I didn't care whether it was a boy or a girl. I wasn't worried about Helen's health or about her running off with the kid. I just savored the moment."

For the entire month of August the McRobbies basked in the euphoria of prospective parenthood. Helen was carrying their baby. *Their baby.* That was all that mattered during those first few weeks as Glenn and Linda slowly absorbed the news of Helen's pregnancy. Elaine called in with occasional progress reports—just often enough to bring the McRobbies down to reality—but otherwise little occurred to distract them from their fantasies. The baby's due date made it imperative that they get the new house finished. As her own general contractor, Linda was spending all her free time at the construction site in the country. This left her little time to dwell on the baby.

Without the house to occupy his every waking moment, Glenn was the first to become aware of how little involvement they had in the physical pregnancy. Although Elaine was good about keeping the McRobbies up to date on Helen's condition, there was little to report during those early months except that she was experiencing some morning sickness. This was just the kind of news every prospective parent wants to hear. But for the McRobbies, who had been so starved for children, it wasn't enough. They missed the tangible evidence of their child's growth. Moreover, as Helen passed through the dangerous first three months, both of the McRobbies feared a miscarriage. They were often tense, worried, apprehensive. It was little wonder that they held back on both emotional involvement and enthusiasm.

It wasn't until Thanksgiving, when Helen came down with the flu, that the McRobbies realized how much they had to lose. For twenty-four hours they lived with the possibility that the fetus was endangered. And suddenly they felt the real force of this baby tugging at their hearts. As terrifying as this incident was, it validated the McRobbie's position as parents in absentia. The baby was now a very live entity. By this point in the pregnancy, they had discovered that surrogate parenting was filled with as much frustration as joy. It was trying to be entirely dependent on the clinic for information on their baby's development. And it was frustrating to have their moods so bound up with the progress of this unseen fetus. A positive report on Helen's condition could send them soaring for days. By the same token, the least negative insinuation from Elaine could plunge them into the depths of depression. But what the McRobbies found most difficult was Elaine's decision in early December to drop her policy of strict anonymity between surrogates and couples.

Elaine had decided that contact between both parties should be optional. Although she would not force them to meet Helen, she felt they should do so at the time of birth. In her opinion, this was a healthier way of experiencing surrogate parenting. Unprepared for this development, the McRobbies spent many hours trying to come to grips with a problem that wasn't at issue when they joined Elaine's program a year earlier. Should they meet their surrogate? How much should they participate in her pregnancy? How much should they participate in the birth? There were no easy answers. The thought of actually meeting Helen and participating in the birth had some appeal. And observing her progress firsthand would certainly be a treat. On the other hand, there was always the possibility that they would dislike her or find her disappointing in some way. And if they did form a relationship, what would happen after the birth? What if they became attached to her and began to feel guilty about asking her to relinquish the baby?

For every positive option the elimination of the anonymity rule offered, it opened up a plethora of moral and ethical issues that left the McRobbies feeling beleaguered, vulnerable, and defenseless. Elaine's gesture, so humanitarian in intent, served only to remind the McRobbies of the risks inherent in surrogate parenting. When all was said and done, they opted to continue with the status quo. Anonymity had presented its frustrations, but it was safe. It neatly defined the roles of surrogate and couple. It was businesslike. But as the mother to be who had hired another woman to do her job, Linda found this decision particularly excruciating. What sort of creep would turn her back on the woman who was carrying her child, she wondered. The answer was simple: one who was terrified of the surrogate's control over the baby.

Helen and the baby were doing well. She had gained a total of nine pounds by December and was well over the nausea she had experienced in the fall. This news—which coincided with the Christmas season—was so exciting that the McRobbies threw themselves into holiday preparations with gusto. There were presents for everyone, including Helen and her little girl. During her many forays to area stores, Linda stifled her urge to buy toys and clothing for the baby. "It was killing me, but I didn't dare," she said. Her instincts told her that they had many hurdles to cross before this baby became a part of their family.

Although the birth was still months away, the McRobbies were surprised to learn at about this time that Elaine was already making preparations. The baby would be born in the city where Helen lived, which was a three-to-four hour drive from the McRobbies' home. They would have the option of participating in the labor or waiting until after Helen had given birth to see the child.

Options, options, and more options. With the change in clinic policy the McRobbies suddenly felt inundated by options. For several weeks they seriously toyed with the idea of being present in the labor room. Under normal circumstances no parent wants to miss the birth of his or her child. But the McRobbies agreed that these weren't normal circumstances. They had begun to realize that in opting for a surrogate birth, they had forfeited much that would ordinarily be considered normal. For example, Glenn, who would not have hesitated to assist Linda in labor, couldn't quite bring himself to witness a strange woman in labor—even a woman who was carrying his child. Linda would have loved to have been the first to hold their baby, but she decided that she didn't want to meet Helen for the first time under those conditions.

In early January they told Elaine they would not attend the labor. They had opted for second best—arriving at the hospital as soon as possible to allow the bonding to take place. Elaine accepted their decision but introduced a disquieting note. It seemed that Helen's little girl was having trouble accepting the fact that Mommy would not be bringing home a little brother or sister from the hospital. She wanted to know whether the McRobbies would furnish the clinic with additional photographs of themselves. Perhaps the pictures would be useful in explaining to Helen's daughter that the baby belonged to someone else. Though slightly unnerved at being dragged into what they felt were Helen's problems, the McRobbies mailed off the pictures. With the move to their new house scheduled for late January, they had little time to worry about the impact of the pregnancy on someone else's child.

On the day before the move Linda chose the wallpaper for the nursery. It was a very special moment for her. She stood in the nursery, a swatch of paper in hand, and shared a very private moment with her future child. She imagined changing the baby, nuzzling its nose, wiping away tears, and playing peekaboo. There were only three months to go. The house the McRobbies moved into was a mess of unfinished rooms and sawdust. But neither of them cared. Suddenly the whole world had awakened to the fact that they were having a baby. Even the workmen who swarmed in and out of the house began to ask about the birth. When a friend of Linda's called to inquire about a gift—the baby's first—she became exultant about everything. And then there were all the showers to think about. Everyone the McRobbies knew seemed to be planning a baby shower for them. Linda's thoughts of and plans for the baby gave her such a feeling of euphoria that in mid-January she was able to look out at the snow-covered landscape and feel that spring was right around the corner. In a burst of ebullience and goodwill, she even wrote to Helen on an impulse to make her a part of it all. "I was so up", she said "that I was even considering whether to keep in touch with her after the birth."

From all appearances the birth promised to be trouble-free. Elaine called early in January to say that they were over the cautionary period. At this stage the fetus was large enough to survive even a premature birth. In fact, Helen seemed to be carrying a very big baby. But she gave everyone a little jolt of fear one day when her car broke down on the highway while she was en route to the clinic for an ultrasound. She was stranded for hours, but although she suffered some cold and fatigue, there were no further complications. Even so, the McRobbies were shaken. They had begged Elaine to make other arrangements so that Helen could be kept off the roads during the winter months. But the director held fast to her rules and insisted that Helen continue her checkups with the physician who was affiliated with the center.

The McRobbies were curious about the baby's sex, and on January 31 they learned that Helen was carrying a four-pound baby boy. Ebullient, carried away with the miracle of it all, Glenn told everyone who would listen about his son. He was a little disappointed for Linda, but she was philosophical about not having a daughter. And like most expectant mothers, her main desire was for a healthy baby. With its gender known, the McRobbies now had the luxury of naming their baby. Actually, a boy's name had been settled months earlier—Bernard Glennon McRobbie, if it was a boy. Bernard after Linda's father, and Glennon for an old family name on Glenn's side.

Well into her third trimester, Helen continued to experience a perfect pregnancy. In the meantime, Linda and Glenn had to overcome yet another obstacle. It had finally dawned on them that they would soon be parents—instant parents without the benefit of a visible pregnancy to break them into the nurturing mold. In all those years during which they had prayed for a child, they had given little thought to what it would mean to actually have one in the house. Diapering, feedings, formulas, and baths were totally foreign to the McRobbies. After spending an entire weekend reading up on infant care, they were more confused than ever. "God, babies are just food-processing machines," Glenn concluded. "I can't believe how much work this is." Even Linda, who was planning to leave her job to care for the baby, found the amount of work the baby involved overwhelming.

Around the end of February Helen wrote to ask how they felt about having a son. She was especially curious about Glenn's reaction. In the same letter she told the McRobbies how active the baby was—so much so that he kept her up almost every night. From her letters, Helen certainly seemed nice, Linda thought. But with the March 30 birth date fast approaching, she couldn't shake the fear that the surrogate mother would insist on keeping the baby. Neither Glenn nor Elaine could convince her that her worries were groundless.

And in the absence of sympathy, Linda directed her growing annoyance over the uncertainties of surrogate parenting at the director. She became increasingly resentful of Elaine's tendencies to change rules abruptly, whether regarding anonymity or finances. Glenn came to share Linda's resentment. With so much money and so many emotions riding on this baby—by now the McRobbies had spent $25,000—Linda wanted more than the "I hope so's" that usually came from Elaine. She and Glenn wanted things to be businesslike and professional.

Although Elaine eventually changed the open-ended aspect of her contract, she did so too late to affect the McRobbies. She also learned too late that her frequent references to Helen's emotional problems only fed the concerns both McRobbies had about the outcome of their surrogate parenting experience. If the McRobbies had ever had any doubts that surrogate parenting would be a risky business, there was none now.

As the months wore on it became clear to Glenn and Linda that Helen was the key to their happiness. Only when she delivered and agreed to sign the baby over to them would the child be theirs. If this aspect of surrogate parenting was known to them before the celebrated "Baby M" case, it did not hit home until Helen was well along in her pregnancy. Thankfully, the baby shower Linda's mother had scheduled for early March came along just in time to deflect a little of the apprehension they were experiencing.

On the day of the party Linda walked into a living room packed with friends, relations, and as many teddy bears as her mother could find. But even this upbeat event had its downside. By the end of the afternoon she had grown tired of fielding questions about surrogate parenting. And she was sick of the subtle reminders that it was another woman, not she, who was carrying her husband's baby.

Though Linda found the shower trying, it did infuse her with renewed spirit. She decided that it was time to buy some baby clothes. And after an afternoon of poking around baby stores, she and Glenn finally settled on a sailor suit. The shopping excursion reasserted Linda's timid optimism that everything would work out.

Yet for every day that she could say things were turning out "real well," there was another when her anxiety over Helen's influence over the baby was overwhelming. Helen had made another request for photographs, and this time the McRobbies said no. To make matters worse, Linda discovered that Glenn had revealed the baby's name in a letter to Helen. She was furious. She didn't think they should do anything to encourage Helen's continued interest in the baby. Linda knew she would never be sure of anything until she and Glenn had the baby safely in their arms and could take him home. But they soon received another letter from Helen—this one describing her physical complaints. Reading about Helen's discomfort was so upsetting that Glenn and Linda took Elaine up on her offer to meet another surrogate mother in the program. Elaine thought it was time they learned something about the surrogate's point of view.

The woman they met was several months behind Helen in her pregnancy. The McRobbies found her gentle and unthreatening. After the encounter Linda was more willing to consider meeting Helen in the hospital. Both she and Glenn now felt more sympathetic to their surrogate and wrote to inquire about the baby.

Plans for the baby's birth were finalized on March 7. The baby would remain in the hospital nursery for forty-eight hours after birth in order to give Glenn and Linda some time to work with the nursing staff on infant care. Helen, in the meantime, wanted to see the baby after he was born and once again before he left the hospital. In light of the pressure she was getting from her boyfriend to keep the child, Elaine thought this arrangement would help her in the relinquishing process. While willing to accept the forty-eight-hour stay in the hospital, both McRobbies felt downright queasy about Helen, her boyfriend, and the prospect of sharing visitation with the surrogate. In her worst moments, Linda imagined that Helen and her boyfriend were plotting to steal the baby. Even Glenn was disturbed by their own lack of control. Or more properly put, by the amount of control Elaine was exerting over the process by allowing Helen access to the baby while in the hospital. More upsetting still was the realization that there was absolutely nothing they could do about it.

At the very least, the days in March were dwindling as quickly as the snowbanks that had buried the McRobbies' new house. One morning in the middle of the month Glenn arrived at work to find the office empty. Someone finally came by and asked if he could check a leaky faucet in the kitchen. When Glenn opened the kitchen door, he was greeted with cheers and congratulations from the entire bank staff. Among the presents he received were a miniature basketball and a baby basketball outfit. He was overcome. This was the first shower anyone had thrown for him. At home he and Linda were working overtime to finish the house before they brought Bernie home. Although the carpenters had finished, they still had to polyurethane the floors, wallpaper, and prepare baby clothes.

In the meantime, reports from Elaine were coming in almost daily now. Except for extreme pelvic pressure, Helen was doing fine. Unfortunately, from the McRobbies' viewpoint, she had not backed down on her request to spend time with the baby in the hospital. In fact, she wanted the freedom to spend as much time with him as she liked. Linda couldn't believe it. "The rules are changing again," she told Glenn before calling Elaine to discuss limiting Helen's visitation rights with the baby. Although Elaine was outwardly sympathetic, she remained adamant that Helen be given access to the baby while the McRobbies were in the hospital. She felt strongly that Helen should be able to spend time with the baby before saying good-bye forever. It was an essential part of the emotional healing process.

Linda hung up feeling desperate and out of control. As the only person in this trio who had no biological connection with Bernie, she felt particularly vulnerable. Once again she was reminded of the uncertainty of the entire surrogate parenting process. There was always an unknown element.

Then the doctor, expecting an early birth, moved the baby's due date up to March 23. The McRobbies were elated. When that day came and went without anything happening, Helen went shopping in an attempt to "jiggle the baby into labor." Their nerves were so taut that a few nights later both Glenn and Linda woke at 3:00 A.M., finding it impossible to get back to sleep They sat up and talked. There was still no baby when the original due date of March 30 passed. By this time the McRobbies were basket cases. Elaine's nightly calls helped, but there was nothing she could do about getting the baby into the world any faster than he intended to arrive. And despite the fact that Helen was miserable, there was no indication that the doctor intended to induce labor.

On April Fool's Day Linda woke tense and upset. Exhausted and on edge from the waiting, she couldn't get it out of her head that Elaine had mistreated them. Convinced that the clinic director had become the surrogate's partisan, she was disturbed that Elaine continued to involve them in Helen's problems with her daughter. What if Helen expected her daughter to form a relationship with Bernie, her biological half brother? Linda wondered. Thoroughly upset with the situation, she called Elaine and demanded to know what was being done about the little girl's expectations. But, as far as Elaine was concerned, the child's curiosity about her half brother was normal "There's no way to control the future," she told Linda, turning a brushfire into a major conflagration. With the birth imminent, the last thing Linda wanted to be reminded of was their lack of control over Bernie's relatives.

"It's all these things—the psychological implications— that I wish I had known about in advance," she complained to Glenn after speaking to Elaine. "I'm angry with her for not making things smoother for us; for making us feel guilty about Helen and her kid. I wish I could go to the hospital and feel secure about what will happen." Glenn didn't feel all that secure either, but he hung on to his belief that they could win in court if Helen gave them trouble over the baby. Although he had retained his buoyant spirits throughout much of the tense recent months, even he professed to be "going nuts" when April crept along without any news.

When the phone rang at 7:30 on the morning of April 4, both Glenn and Linda nearly killed each other rushing to get it. But it was another false alarm—just the carpenter calling to check on the back door. By now the phone was ringing day and night with friends and relatives who were as anxious about the birth as they were. But Elaine still had no news. A few days later she called to say that Helen was dilated to two centimeters and it appeared that things would progress without undue delay. So much for that report. Within twenty-four hours the baby, though it had calmed down, was kicking wildly again. The doctor was talking about inducing labor if nothing happened within the week.

Could Glenn and Linda wait that long? They had no choice, so they settled down to seven more days of tension and anxiety. After waiting this long for a child, Glenn figured they could wait some more. He was hoping, however, that the baby would arrive in time for his own birthday on April 11. When four more days passed without any news, the McRobbies pretty much gave up the constant phone vigils. Too exhausted to worry any longer, they wallpapered the nursery and generally went about their business as best they could.

Helen, however, had no such options. Feeling as if she was going to burst, she took a bumpy ride on April 8 in the hope of inducing labor. She even raked leaves for good measure. And still no baby came. Elaine phoned that night to tell the McRobbies that nothing had happened yet. They went to bed feeling tired of the whole thing. Before she fell asleep, Linda wondered for a long time how ready she was for motherhood. Sometimes she felt prepared; at other times she simply didn't know.

The next morning Elaine phoned the McRobbies with the thrilling news that they were finally parents. A week after Bernie's birth, in the sun-filled warmth of their bedroom, Linda and Glenn took turns holding their tiny son. At that moment, with the soft light from the windows bathing everything in radiance, no one could have guessed at the years of trauma and heartache that preceded this birth. No one could have guessed that Bernie McRobbie had not come into the world in the usual way.

# 4 | Couples: A Nationwide Perspective

From the media coverage it would seem that couples who seek the services of surrogate parenting clinics are very much like Glenn and Linda McRobbie—professional people in their late thirties with higher than average incomes. After surveying surrogate parenting clinics nationwide it became clear that, in fact, their clients come from a variety of cultural and economic backgrounds. It is just as common to find a steelworker seeking the services of a surrogate parenting clinic as it is to find a lawyer. (And it is becoming increasingly common to find clinics serving clients from Europe and the Orient.)

What is different about these couples—what sets them apart from other couples who happen to be infertile—is a driving need to have a child. Theirs is a need so deep, so intense, that they are willing to pay almost any price, take any risk, and suffer just about any inconvenience or emotional strain to make that dream come true.

Like the McRobbies, most of these couples will tell you

that money is no object. Some have even taken out second or third mortgages on their homes to pay the hefty surrogate parenting fees, which by early 1987 ranged from $15,000 to $40,000. (At that time most couples were paying between $15,000 and $30,000). Despite the financial cost and difficulty of being involved in a procedure so experimental that no one knows how the outcome will affect the marriage, the family, or the child twenty years hence, very few of the couples interviewed for this book had any sense of being reproductive pioneers. For couples this desperate to have children, surrogate parenting does not exist on the fringes of reproductive science. It is their only means of producing that precious child they feel is a necessary component of their lives. "We wouldn't have done this if we could easily have had natural children," explained an infertile adoptive mother from Massachusetts who had had one child through natural means before developing fertility problems. She now believes that she will never be able to bear another child of her own and must depend on surrogate mothers for additional children.

Couples who did have a sense of being involved in something very new, very different, and somewhat daring were in the minority. However, many couples surveyed had come under criticism from their families or society for their actions. As a result, of the thirty-four couples interviewed for this book, the majority agreed to talk about their experiences only if they could do so anonymously. But whether or not they were open about their involvement in surrogate parenting, statistics show that these couples are being joined by increasing numbers in their decision to pursue this alternative.

Since 1980 an estimated 12,000 to 15,000 infertile couples have contacted surrogate parenting clinics nationwide. Of these, clinic directors had accepted about 1,000 into their programs by early 1987. There had been about 600 clinic births as of that date. Based on these figures, it may be expected that at least 1,000 couples and 2,000 surrogates will soon be joining clinic programs annually, experts say. The couples who agreed to talk about the impact of surrogate parenting on their lives came from Arkansas, California, Colorado, Florida, Kansas, Massachusetts, Oregon, Texas, Vermont, and the state of Washington. Of these one-third were Californians. All but one couple had taken part in an organized surrogate parenting program. A number of the couples—especially those from the South and the Southwest—had even traveled to clinics in California and Kansas because there were no facilities in their part of the country.

Although they were not queried directly about their religious and socioeconomic backgrounds, many couples volunteered information that indicates that they are a varied lot. They range from blue-collar workers to the upper reaches of the economic elite. Given the regional spread and economic/cultural differences represented, one might expect these couples to hold wide-ranging attitudes about surrogate parenting. This was not the case. Whatever their individual religious or political beliefs, they all shared a deep support for surrogate parenting. What surrogate parenting has given them is a control over the childbearing process that their infertility had denied them—control so precious that despite scattered concerns about finances and the impact of this procedure on their child, not one couple interviewed advocated even a temporary ban on the process in order to allow medical or ethical experts to study its implications. "No ban!" wrote many in the margins of their survey forms.

The clinics and their cadres of lawyers, doctors, and psychologists appeared to play a major role in shaping attitudes. This is true of their impact on the couples and surrogates in their programs as well as of the role they have played in shaping national opinion about surrogate parenting. What attitudinal differences did emerge from this informal study were closely linked to the indoctrination the couples received from surrogate parenting clinics. For example, couples that favored anonymity tended to go to clinics or centers that foster anonymity between the couple and the surrogate. Similarly, those who favored contact tended to go to clinics that foster contact between couples and surrogates. Clinics with a more avant-garde approach to surrogate parenting—for example, those that encourage joint participation in the birth process—are located mainly on the West Coast. Centers on the East Coast and those in the Midwest tended to be somewhat more conservative.

In addition to voicing wholehearted support of the procedure, the couples interviewed were also united in their feelings of frustration with the adoption process. In their dealings with adoption agencies, most of them had suffered experiences as harrowing as those reported by the McRobbies. And, as infertile couples, they face a shrinking pool of healthy, domestic babies. For that reason, it's not surprising that the decision to forgo adoption dominated the list of reasons these couples gave for turning to surrogate parenting. It eliminates the years of waiting for a child only to be told that there is no baby available or that they are not acceptable parents.

Equally important to these couples was the chance to have as much genetic input into the process as possible. Although surrogate parenting involves only the husband's genes, many couples found this infinitely preferable to having no genetic link at all with their prospective child. Feminists have criticized this aspect of surrogate parenting, dismissing it as a process designed to satisfy the man's chauvinistic need for a genetic heir. But the majority of wives interviewed were found to be just as eager as their husbands for a child that was at least partially theirs genetically.

The majority of couples surveyed pointed out that for them surrogate parenting was the only viable option. For many adoption had either failed or had proved to be undesirable, and in vitro fertilization—in which the wife's egg is fertilized by the husband's sperm in the laboratory and then implanted in the woman's uterus—was not possible. "We wanted a kid and I couldn't have one," a Florida adoptive mother said of her and her husband's decision to try surrogate parenting. "This was the next best thing to in vitro fertilization, and it's better than adoption. At least we know about the mother's background." Another adoptive mother from Massachusetts said she and her husband chose surrogate parenting because it offered both genetic benefits and time benefits. "We didn't have to wait the five to seven years it would take for an adoption to go through," she asserted.

For about one-fifth of those surveyed, surrogate parenting was the number-one choice of alternatives because it offered them some personal involvement in the creation of their child. Other, secondary reasons found to be instrumental in many couples' decision to select this method include the fact that surrogate parenting allowed a husband to have a child of his own; it created a natural sibling for an existing child; and it gave couples firsthand knowledge of the natural mother or at least access to her biological records.

Nancy and Carl Martin of Port Townsend, Washington were among the few couples who sought out surrogate parenting as a means of producing a child in a second marriage. Nancy has two children from a previous marriage, after which she suffered tubal pregnancies and was told that she should not attempt any others. The Martins were in the process of adopting a Korean child in 1978 when they learned of Noel Keane's Detroit clinic and decided to give it a try. Carl Martin, who was then employed as a heavy-equipment operator, worked overtime to finance the surrogate parenting fees. Their son was born in December 1981. "I felt that if I could let my husband have a biological child, I should," said Nancy. "It was an experience I had already had. I felt I was giving him something I wasn't able to do myself." The

Martins' experience has been a positive one. Their son was five when they responded to the survey, and by all reports he is doing fine.

How well couples cope with the surrogate parenting process appears to depend on both their emotional makeup and that of the surrogate mother, the program they choose, the attitude of friends, family, and coworkers, and on the general atmosphere of the community in which they live. The majority of couples surveyed reported having had extremely favorable experiences with surrogate parenting—experiences that were for the most part far less trying than those the McRobbies lived through. For the McRobbies the anonymity issue, the risks, and Linda McRobbie's fears about the surrogate's motives all combined to make the process a difficult one. Although they are thrilled with their son, it is doubtful that either of the McRobbies would echo the sentiments of an Oregon couple, who described their surrogate parenting experience as being magical from start to finish.

Although they are in a minority, the McRobbies were not the only couple to experience problems with the surrogate parenting process. About one-fourth of those surveyed found the pregnancy period difficult, and several reported that they had trouble working with their surrogates. The couples who had the most difficult time seem to be those who thought of surrogate parenting as an activity on the fringe of acceptability. They were anxious about their actions and consequently less willing to talk openly about their experiences lest they expose themselves and their child. On the other hand, couples who attended programs in which openness was encouraged seemed to exhibit very little self-consciousness about their involvement in surrogate parenting. They seemed content about what they had done and happier with the outcome. It should be noted that many of these couples live on the West coast, where experimental procedures such as surrogate parenting thrive openly. (Although California clinics have spearheaded the development of therapeutic approaches to assist surrogates and couples in better coping with their surrogate parenting experiences, they are not alone in their therapeutic approach. And they are not alone in their success.)

In the end the survey found both couples who extolled the virtues of the surrogate parenting process and could sing its praises purely and without reservations and those who lamented what they thought to be the program's natural shortcomings. A Massachusetts adoptive mother said of the outcome of her experience with surrogate parenting, "It was wonderful. The process was unnecessarily draining. We didn't know in the end that the delivery and the hospital would go as smoothly as it did. We hadn't spoken to anyone who could reassure us." Said another adoptive mother of the process: "It took a lot of getting used to. I wasn't supportive of the surrogate in the beginning. I didn't really know what to say to this woman."

An adoptive mother from Florida got to know her surrogate mother so well that the two of them often lunched together. In this way she was able to experience the pregnancy, which she thoroughly enjoyed. Difficulties later arose in the hospital, though, when this particular surrogate mother wanted to nurse the baby. "I found it upsetting because I couldn't do it," the adoptive mother related. "Then the surrogate cried when she had to give the baby up, which was hard on me. I was glad when she moved out of state."

Despite such problems, many of the couples interviewed are considering having other children with the assistance of a surrogate mother. Some even hope they will be able to use the same surrogate. In many ways they are much like women who have suffered a painful labor: within a month of the baby's arrival, they had forgotten the pain and were willing to do it all over again. Couples who had problems with the procedure agreed that it helps to know what to expect. There was also a general agreement that it was best to be enrolled in programs in which the directors are schooled in the specific problems that can affect adoptive couples. Couples involved in these programs generally handled surrogacy better than those who were given little or no guidance.

Surrogate parenting has become sufficiently wide-spread—especially in California—for service personnel to be able to isolate the difficulties common to many couples. Clinic directors and psychologists who work with adoptive couples in a surrogate parenting setting have begun to target these problems for counseling purposes. They agree that much of the trauma couples encounter as part of the surrogacy process is both predictable and preventable. For example, there is an emerging consensus among professionals in the field that couples should resolve the emotional issues surrounding their infertility before embarking on a surrogate parenting course. They also agree that both husband and wife must be mutually interested in the process. The fear that the surrogate mother will renege on her terms of the contract and want to keep the baby is now widely recognized, as is the understanding that couples may need some assistance in adjusting to parenthood. And professionals in the field also realize that most couples in their programs need guidance in dealing with the difficult issue of what to tell their child about his or her natural mother when the times comes.

The couples interviewed for this survey encountered some problems as a team while other issues were found to be sex related or role related. Husbands, for example, often worried about their potency around insemination time, while their wives—the adoptive mothers—often experienced some jealousy and pain at the realization that they were turning to other women to do their job. Hilary Hanafin, the staff psychologist at the Center of Surrogate Parenting in Los Angeles, has counseled many surrogates and couples since she became involved with surrogate parenting in 1983. When a prospective couple first comes to her center she is particularly keen on ensuring that they have come for the right reason. The right reason, Hanafin feels, is that they both want a child and are both willing to make the emotional and financial sacrifices necessary to have that child.

Too often, though, Hanafin has seen couples enter the surrogate parenting program motivated by guilt or by the need to make one or the other spouse happy at the expense of their own happiness. When couples are motivated by the wrong reasons, Hanafin believes it is unlikely the situation will work out. "I see infertile women whose guilt about their infertility is so great that they're willing to use a surrogate mother to make their husbands happy," she said. "I've also seen husbands whose needs to have their genes represented are so strong that they'll go to a program no matter how their wives feel." Ideally, she believes, a couple should enter a surrogate parenting program as a team. They should both want to be there. She also feels it is important for a couple to explore who wants the process and why. Although some couples are capable of working out this extremely sensitive issue on their own, for many the question of whether or not to become involved with a surrogate mother can be tense and difficult. But whether by themselves or through infertility counseling, she believes this is a crucial step in alleviating future problems.

Hanafin has found that both surrogate mothers and couples often deny their real feelings. "Denial," she said "is a very sophisticated coping mechanism, and is clearly seen as an active way of dealing with the [infertility] problem." In order for surrogate parenting to work well for a couple, Hanafin believes they must be comfortable with their infertility—comfortable enough to allow a third party to enter into their marriage. She also feels strongly that programs that encourage anonymity between surrogate mothers and couples allow the couple to deny their infertility. They make it easier for the couple "not to confront the issue of their infertility head-on. Drop the anonymity," she counsels, "and then you do have to confront it".

Although Hanafin feels that it is healthier for couples not to deny the surrogate, she also recognizes that it is natural for them to feel this way. She therefore advises couples to work with their infertility to the point where they can acknowledge it. She does sanction anonymity for couples who cannot overcome their discomfort with the surrogate, but she feels adjustment becomes harder for the child whose parents have denied the surrogate. They're more likely to be parents who are handicapped by their inability to deal with the knowledge of a third party openly and honestly.

Once a couple has wrestled with the issue of their infertility and settled on surrogate parenting as the answer to their childbearing problems, Hanafin believes they can more successfully deal with society at large. But she concedes that the task is not an easy one for all that. Couples must struggle with "the fact that society doesn't know how to deal with them." And they must also understand "that people unfamiliar with surrogate parenting just don't know how to react to the news that a friend, family member, or coworker has hired a strange woman to bear their child."

Do you throw a baby shower for an adoptive mother? Whom do you tell about the surrogacy, and how do you respond to their negative comments? These are just a few of the more mundane issues that infertile couples who choose surrogate parenting must resolve during the course of the pregnancy. According to Hanafin, "Coping with the rest of the world's naïveté and judgmental attitude can be a real struggle. I tell people that older children, selected members of the extended family, and close friends should know the truth. They can tell others that the child is adopted, which minimizes the controversial part. The family," she said, "is usually very accepting, curious, sometimes anxious, but ultimately positive. Most of our couples have had a lot of support."

Although husbands can have problems dealing with surrogate parenting—mostly during the artificial insemination process and at the time of birth—psychologists have found that the burden of adjustment usually rests on the adoptive mother. Most difficult for these women, it has been found, is finding a place for themselves in a process in which someone else has assumed their natural role. Hanafin works hard in helping adoptive mothers "establish a role despite their lack of a biological contribution." At the Center of Surrogate Parenting, she encourages adoptive mothers to "literally participate in the conception and insemination process, including the doctor's visits". She has concluded that "the adoptive mother has a place in surrogate parenting, but she has to create it and feel comfortable with it".

Hanafin believes the adoptive mother plays the most crucial psychological role in the triangle made up of husband, wife, and surrogate mother. The bond between the two women is often the source of the surrogate's emotional satisfaction. Often they can't wait to place the baby in the arms of the infertile woman." What happens to that bonding between the two women after the birth? When there is anonymity both the couple and the surrogate simply resume their former lives. And although they may have been greatly altered by the surrogacy experience, severing the surrogate parenting tie is not an issue they must confront directly.

On the other hand, when emotional ties have been established between the two parties, the whole postpartum question becomes far more complicated. Some couples remain close friends with the woman who bore their child, even to the point of including the surrogate in the child's upbringing. But more commonly, the contact remains high for several months after birth and then dwindles until it is marked only by a card sent on birthdays and at Christmas or by an occasional phone call.

Whatever the couple decides to do about contact with their surrogate mother after the birth, Hanafin feels that they are bound to suffer some guilt. Couples, according to Hanafin, usually feel indebted on the one hand while on the other, part of them wishes she would go away and that they never had to resort to hiring a surrogate mother. "We try to acknowledge these feelings," said Hanafin, but insist that "the couple can't ignore the surrogate. Most couples are sophisticated enough to at least go through the motions and break off contact two months after birth."

Even couples who maintain minimal contact with the surrogate mother must at some time cope with the problem of what to tell their child about his or her biological mother. Hanafin counsels a policy of "straightforward openness and honesty as soon as the child begins to ask questions." For very young children she advises parents to tell them something like, "Mommy's tummy was broken and we had to have a special lady help us." Hanafin further suggests that couples, make the word adoption a household word so that the child first hears it from them." As the child gets older and the questions become more sophisticated, she maintains, the answers can become more sophisticated.

Lynn Brown, the administrative coordinator at the Center for Reproductive Alternatives in Pleasant Hills, California, says that her clinic works closely with couples as well as surrogates. She and her colleagues—Bruce Rappaport, director, and Marty Sochet, staff psychologist—believe the adoptive couple need just as much reassurance and support as the surrogate mother. In fact, of the clinics surveyed for this book this center was among the few that were found to operate a separate counseling group for couples. Kathryn Wyckoff of the Center for Reproductive Alternatives in San Clemente, California, also runs such a group.

At the northern California center that Brown administers, all couples are expected to attend group therapy as soon as they are accepted into the surrogate parenting program. The group has become so popular that some people go just for the social aspect. Others go for support—especially during the periods of waiting that can make surrogate parenting so excruciating for the couple. Brown and Sochet counsel everyone in their program, including the surrogate mothers, that surrogacy takes time. "They [the couples] always feel it's not moving ahead fast enough. Everyone wants it to happen five years ago," Brown said. "But we must take the time to make sure all the legal, medical, and financial things are taken care of to avoid disaster later on. Sometimes couples will demand more than one match meeting, then things seem to stand still and everyone goes crazy." According to Brown, the insemination period is often the most difficult for many couples. Things become more difficult, still, when the surrogate has problems conceiving. "The natural father may have questions about his own fertility," she said, "and insemination for him can be degrading and embarrassing."

Resolution of infertility issues is equally important at the Center for Reproductive Alternatives as at Hanafin's Center of Surrogate Parenting in Los Angeles. "We don't want couples who haven't accepted their infertility. If they aren't accepting of their situation, it's possible for them to go through really bad problems," said Brown. She also takes special pains to assist the adoptive mother through the surrogate parenting process, convinced that the infertile woman too often blames herself for the expense of the program—a financial drain that would not be necessary if she were fertile. "Usually the surrogates are much younger and more outgoing, which can create jealousy issues," Brown added. "If we sense that this is the case, we recommend that they seek outside counseling before joining the program."

The last thing Brown wants is for her program to "lead some couple to divorce." She also refuses to accept a couple when she senses that one spouse is going along with surrogacy just to make the other happy. "That won't work," she said. "The surrogate will be unhappy; the marriage will be unhappy." The Center for Reproductive Alternatives is also extremely insistent on contact between couples and their surrogates. In fact, no couple who refuse to at least meet the woman who will bear their child is accepted into the program. Those who prefer partial anonymity are allowed to deal with their surrogate mother on a first-name basis only.

However, the clinic insists that they spend time together. Brown believes that when people want to deal in secrecy it is a sure sign that they haven't dealt with their infertility. "They want a cure without dealing with the issues," she said. For some couples anonymity can be a convenient form of self-protection, a need Brown feels tends to disappear after they meet their surrogate.

It has been Brown's experience that contact between couples and surrogates also minimizes the one, major fear that all infertile couples share: the terror that the surrogate mother will want to keep the baby. She argues that once they get to know each other there is very little fear of this. "It literally becomes teamwork," she said. "Then it's the couple's child, not the surrogate's." Although fear of the surrogate is difficult to work with and has been found to be groundless in most cases, Brown understands the couples' feelings. With all the negative publicity generated by the "Baby M" case, she feels it would be surprising if couples weren't anxious. But there are other factors that feed the trauma and tension of having a child via a surrogate mother.

Brown points out that, like the McRobbies, many couples enter surrogacy after waging a draining battle with infertility. Many of them have also faced rejection by adoption agencies or had natural mothers decide to keep the babies at the final hour of adoption. Such experiences, she believes, often make couples initially indifferent to the risks inherent in surrogate parenting. They just want to forge ahead with pregnancy. As they become more involved in the procedure, however, and more concerned about the baby's fate, anxiety over the surrogate mother's intent usually increases. Fortunately, according to Brown, couples at the Center for Reproductive Alternatives can take their concerns to a support group. Most couples, Brown feels, have found their fears and anxieties surrounding the surrogate's relinquishment of the child less threatening after attending these support-group sessions.

The group has also been useful for discussing both the birth and the subsequent adoption process. Brown says that in these sessions couples often talk about what can be expected from the social worker and the courts. They talk about how the birth and having a child will affect their relationship, and they even discuss child rearing and who will assume the burden. She has seen cases in which the husband worried about how to handle the fact that someone other than his wife was bearing his child. In some instances neither the husband nor the wife knew how to deal with the birth. It was then that contact with other couples proved to be most valuable. "They hear from other couples that it worked out—couples who were in the delivery room. The apprehension has to do with the unknown," Brown said.

A number of the couples interviewed for this book—couples who did not participate in the two programs discussed—wish their program had offered some sort of counseling/support group. It would have been nice, they reported after the fact, to have been able to talk to other couples in a therapeutic setting about many of the frustrations and anxieties inherent in the process. According to these couples their biggest dilemmas concerned their relationship with the surrogate mother, the fears surrounding her relinquishment of the baby, and, finally, the best way of terminating the relationship with the surrogate. Although most of them also had financial and legal worries, these occupied a secondary position in relation to the emotional issues.

As clinic directors and psychologists have suggested, many of the couples who make contact with their surrogate mothers seem happier than those who decided to maintain full anonymity or had little or no contact. During the surrogate parenting process, these couples also expressed fewer concerns about whether their surrogate mothers would relinquish the child. One drawback to this approach, however, is the development of a relationship that both parties might find difficult to terminate after the birth. Some couples are comfortable maintaining a relationship with their surrogate. If this is not the case, clinic directors advise couples to outline the kind of contact they want from the outset.

Half of the couples who met their surrogate mothers at the beginning of the procedure reported being glad they had done so. The same was found to be true of the couples who came into contact with their surrogate at the time of birth. By contrast, couples who maintained full anonymity were divided on the issue: some had no desire ever to meet their surrogate mother; others regretted not having done so.

"The biggest fear after the birth was that the surrogate might change her mind and come looking for us," said one adoptive mother who chose to maintain complete anonymity. This woman enjoyed the anonymity and explained that she and her husband wanted control over the process because it seemed easier emotionally. Another couple, who met their surrogate mother for the first time in the hospital, reported feeling grateful for the encounter. "We felt somewhat anxious about whether or not she would give up the baby, but it felt good to get acquainted," they acknowledged. Nancy Martin has chosen to get to know her surrogate mother, whom she calls Joyce. "I got to know her very well," she said. "And for me that was wonderful. I don't know how it would work for others, but I sense that if you can't trust your surrogate mother, you shouldn't be doing this."

Although psychologists are convinced that unless surrogate parenting is legalized all couples will have some fears about the relinquishment, there are couples, like the Martins, who claimed they had no such concerns. "That the surrogate mother wouldn't give up the baby never crossed my mind," related another couple who asked not to be identified. But like Glenn McRobbie, others were prepared to wage a custody battle and assumed they would be the winners. Even the Martins discussed what they would do if their surrogate wouldn't give up the child. They decided against a custody battle. "Still, I had three children in my home," said Nancy Martin. "Probably we would have gone for the fight if we were childless. I'm sure my husband would have wanted visitation rights."

In cases where there has been a fear of the surrogate, clinic directors and psychologists have usually found the adoptive mother to be the one who harbored the most concern. The survey conducted for this book confirmed their contention. About one-fourth of these couples reported being afraid that their surrogate would not give up the child. Many of these couples indicated that the wives were more concerned about this happening than their husbands.

Once the child has been born and the surrogate mother has willingly signed him or her over to the adoptive parents, most couples walk straight into the issue of what to tell their child about his or her origins. As with adoption, almost all psychologists urge parents involved in surrogate parenting to be honest with their children about the role a surrogate mother has played in their birth. Dennis Michael Harrison, a forensic psychologist and surrogate parenting consultant from Maryland, said that it is "important for parents to be able to talk to the child about the situation. As in adoption," he noted, "there can be no deceit or secrets. The last thing you want is for an adopted child or a surrogate child to find out accidentally." (*The New York Times,* December 8, 1986.)

Almost all of the couples interviewed for this book said they would tell their children everything they wanted to know about their biological mother. Some were prepared to show their children photographs of the natural mother, and a handful even claimed to be willing to arrange a meeting if this was what the child wanted. "We're going to tell him the truth when the time is right," said one couple. "We'll tell him all the details. It's good to be up-front. In adoptions they're always wondering who the mother is. Our child won't have those questions."

Of all the couples interviewed, only the Martins had a

child old enough to begin asking about his birth. "He has asked for pictures of her and they've been sent," said Nancy Martin, who also included photographs of the surrogate's family in the child's baby book so that he would know they were his relatives. The Martins have assumed that their son will want to know more about his biological mother as he approaches adolescence. "We're prepared for difficult times," Nancy said. "I'm just glad our surrogate has seen him and cares about him. We figure that basically he'll want to know. And we've felt from the beginning that if we were open it wouldn't be a mystery or a dark secret."

How much contact the surrogate and child will eventually have over the years appears to have a lot to do with the relationship the couple has developed with their surrogate mother. Most of the couples interviewed stayed in touch with the surrogate via phone and the mail for several months after birth. Within a year or so, however, one-third of those surveyed reported a decrease of contact. There were several couples who had become friends with their surrogate mothers on a social basis. For instance, Brown has a surrogate and couple in her program who travel on the lecture circuit together.

Dr. Harrison, the Maryland psychologist, doesn't encourage openness between couples and surrogates. Nor does he encourage a continuing relationship. Harrison has said that as in an adoption, "a child needs one set of parents, not Parent Number One and Parent Number Two." And although the Martins maintain close contact with their surrogate, Nancy Martin agrees with Harrison about helping the child sort out his parentage. "This wasn't intended to be two families," she said. "The surrogate is not and hasn't been involved in any of the decision making. She's just another person who cares for him. But there aren't two mothers in the sense that there are two people making decisions about his life."

Despite the issues surrounding contact with surrogates

and what to tell the children, very few of the couples surveyed seemed concerned about the effect of surrogate birth on their child. Two-thirds of the couples surveyed didn't think there would be any negative impact on their child. Like the Martins, they felt that a solid, loving home life would compensate for the fact that a third party had been brought in to conceive and carry the baby. "I don't worry about what's to be," Nancy Martin said. "If you love and nurture a child, he'll be a healthy person. Kids can live with all kinds of adversity if you build their self-esteem."

Although they are in a minority, there are some couples who worry that being the product of a surrogate birth may present difficulties for their child. Two couples have admitted that they have fears for their child. About one-third of the sample surveyed had mixed feelings about how their children would later cope with the knowledge of their birth via surrogacy. "I worry about whether my daughter will feel abandoned by her natural mother," confided one adoptive mother. "Because of the nature of our surrogate parenting program, the natural mother was never in the picture. But I'm not sure the baby will see it that way. I hope that she will be able to understand and that we will be able to answer her questions and tell her it that it was a wonderful thing her surrogate mother did."

Couples tended to be more vocal about the financial aspects of surrogate parenting than about more emotional issues. Although almost 100 percent were in favor of offering some payment for services, complaints about the amount paid to clinics, lawyers, and, in some cases, doctors, were common. A quarter of those surveyed felt that fees charged by the clinic should have been reduced; half of them said the entire process should be cheaper. Some couples suggested that clinics operate on a nonprofit basis like adoption agencies, so—as one couple put it—"they can't take advantage of our misfortune." Complaints aside, no one begrudged the surrogate mother her fee. In fact, one-fifth of those surveyed argued that she should be paid more for her services. "I approve of the surrogate being paid, and even possibly more than she was, but I don't think the clinic should be a profit-making agency," said one father. "It should run like an adoption agency. I know of adoption agencies that charge $5,000 and feed the money back into the system."

There were those, however, who supported the operation of clinics for profit. "Who would do it for nothing?" asked one couple. "We think the money end of it is fine. In a capitalist venture you have to pay for services." Another couple agreed. "It's expensive, but private adoption is pretty expensive too. Some charge $17,000. What's another $4,000 to know where the kid's coming from and have half of it be yours?"

Altering the financial arrangement between the couples and the clinics was just one of a number of suggestions couples offered for improving the surrogate parenting process. Although most of the couples involved in surrogate parenting were found to be staunch advocates of surrogacy, they were not uncritical advocates. There was an almost unanimous agreement that some sort of general regulation of the process, with one-third of the couples supporting legalization of surrogate parenting on a state-by-state or nationwide basis. Although those from California were unanimous in their support of legalization, licensing and government regulation, they had less to say about the nature of specific controls they would support than did couples from other parts of the country. These recommendations included the following: standardization of fees and regulations for operating clinics nationwide; legalization of payment of the surrogate's fee in states where this is outlawed; making the adoptive mother the legal mother at the time of conception; regulating surrogate parenting like adoption; and giving the father automatic custody. There were couples, though, who considered "controls" and "regulations" dirty words. They didn't want to risk implementing any form of government regulation that would affect surrogate parenting.

One-third of those surveyed wanted no control of any kind, not even legalization. "If people feel good about doing this, why should someone step in and stop it?" asked one couple. "People like us don't have a lot of options." An adoptive mother added, "Some people have choices. They can get pregnant. Then there are those who don't. I see surrogate parenting as a viable option. There's no reason to ban it—especially when they could make laws to protect the parties involved. It could just be another contract."

Nancy Martin concluded: "I keep coming back to the fact that we're trying to build families at a time when the family has lost focus. "Let's concentrate on what's right in this process. With divorce and what's going on with the family in twenty years, this is really sad. Society ought to give people credit for wanting to be a family at a time when it doesn't look appealing."

# 2
## THE SURROGATES

# 5 | Tale of a Surrogate Mother

If the Madonna made an appearance in the twentieth century she would probably look a lot like Jane Woodman. With her warm brown eyes, beatific smile, and gentle demeanor, Jane is about as close to the personification of motherhood as you can get. And she doesn't simply look the part; she acts it. Children have always been central to Jane's life. She initially sacrificed a career in nursing education rather than end up childless. But the birth of two girls could not save a loveless marriage. Jane went through a wrenching divorce, earned a nursing degree, and discovered that she could support her family on her own. For many women two children would have been enough—not to mention the prospect of raising them without a husband—but Jane had always wanted a large family. If she had remained married, she had planned to have at least five. She had always found bearing children and caring for them spiritually intoxicating. The thought that the divorce had sabotaged her most enduring dream was far more distressing to Jane than the breakup of her marriage. Would she be able to find another man to bear her children before she became too old? At thirty-six this was a real dilemma for her. It seemed all the odds were against her if having another baby was to coincide with matrimony.

Jane was well aware that many women today become mothers with the help of artificial insemination or the willing participation of a male who does not act as the father. But she rejected this route because it was financially unfeasible. Between her nurse's salary and what she collected in child support, there was barely enough money for her and the two girls, let alone another child. Then another option—less appealing but intriguing, nonetheless—opened to her. Jane discovered that she could be a surrogate mother. What might seem strange and even slightly repugnant to many women was fascinating to her. Although she now dresses conservatively and lives a middle-class existence, Jane still espouses much of the philosophy she embraced during her years as part of the hippie counterculture. Her willingness to share material goods with others, her fascination with Eastern culture and holistic medicine, and her open-minded acceptance of the new and bizarre are all legacies of her past.

If you want to find aging hippies in Massachusetts, you don't go to Cambridge. You go to the section of the Connecticut River Valley where Jane lives. There you can still find communes, with resident potters, carpenters, and organic-vegetable gardeners. There, too, you will find an accepting environment for alternative life-styles. To Jane and many of her associates, the concept of surrogate parenting is altruistic and therefore worthy of consideration. Couple this attitude with Jane's caring nature, her love for children, and a fairly unorthodox approach to life, and you have a natural candidate for the role of surrogate mother. Add to this the fact that she comes from a good family, attended Vassar College for a brief time and has a college degree, and Jane becomes pretty appealing to an infertile couple in search of a stranger to bear their child.

Jane's involvement with surrogate motherhood came about one spring day in 1985 while she was packing to move to the brown-shingled bungalow she had bought with her parents' help. Tired from her efforts, she took a moment to sit at the kitchen table and look out at the lilac bushes in bloom. The children were outside playing and, for once, the house was quiet. Jane picked up an alternative newspaper that circulated in her area and began to browse through it. A year earlier she wouldn't have had the luxury of relaxing in her kitchen. With the divorce, nursing school, and raising two little girls, she didn't even have time for a social life. At the start of her career in nursing only nighttime shifts were available. Eventually her hours became normal. The dream of a house became a reality, and she had even begun to date a little. She wasn't exactly desperate. But as she leafed through the tabloid, an article on a New England surrogate parenting center caught her eye. For the first time Jane realized that there were women—women just like her in Massachusetts—who were bearing children for infertile couples. And they were being paid up to $10,000 for their services.

Jane read every word of the article and then read the whole thing again. She couldn't put the paper down. The notion of bearing a child for an infertile couple both intrigued and repelled her. There had to be an easier, more desirable way to earn $10,000. And with two children, a house, and her new job in the maternity ward of the local hospital, she hardly needed another challenge. Or did she? As much as Jane tried to squelch the idea, the thought of becoming a surrogate mother haunted her. She wondered if this might not be a way of saying thank you for the birth of her own children. For she had known, firsthand, the fear of infertility. After having trouble conceiving her first child she had consulted a Chinese doctor in Boston. He gave her some special Chinese herbs, and soon after taking them she had become pregnant.

Several days passed, and Jane found she couldn't suppress her curiosity any longer. She gave in to the urge to call the surrogate parenting center. A young-sounding woman—Elaine Silver, the director—answered the phone. She and Jane established an immediate rapport. Jane liked Elaine's feminist bent and felt only wholehearted support for her humanitarian goal of finding women to bear children for infertile couples. But when Elaine invited her to visit the clinic, Jane balked. It was one thing to fantasize about surrogacy and quite another to actually allow someone to inseminate her with a stranger's sperm and then live through the pregnancy and birth. There were her children to consider, and the move. . . . She realized that the timing was off. She would just have to wait for her inner voice to tell her when the timing was right.

"I wish-washed back and forth on it and then I finally saw that I didn't want to look back and say to myself, 'I wish I had done that,' " she said of that period in May and June when she was trying to make up her mind whether to be a surrogate mother. "I get these urges that aren't always rational, and I'm glad I've followed them. When I haven't, I've regretted it." As soon as Jane decided to put off the decision, she found herself yearning to have a child again. But it wasn't until Elaine applied a little pressure that she finally agreed to be a surrogate mother. Jane vividly remembers that warm June day. It wasn't the first time Elaine had asked her to work for her. "I guess so," she had told Elaine, putting her off. But on this particular day there was a bit of urgency in Elaine's voice, a little push, that Jane hadn't experienced before.

When Jane gave her the usual "I guess so," Elaine replied, "Well, if you're thinking of doing it, let's get going. Come down to the clinic and see the psychologist and gynecologist." As it turned out, Elaine had a couple in mind for Jane. They were professionals, very family oriented, and they had been trying unsuccessfully for a number of years to have a second child. According to Elaine, they had suffered a great deal of pain over their inability to produce a sibling for their little girl. Jane, who had been leaning toward surrogacy, was hooked by Elaine's description of a couple in need. She didn't feel she could turn back now. "I immediately felt I knew them. I felt I had a connection," she recalled. "Then I felt like it was already decided. I almost felt like it would be betraying a good friend to say no."

Panic set in the minute she hung up the phone, however. The enormity of what she was getting into struck Jane with gut-wrenching fear. "I haven't signed anything," she told herself, trying to calm down. "Nothing has to happen." But it already had. She confided her plans to a few close friends before visiting the clinic for the first time. Some were extremely supportive of her, while others told her that she would hurt her daughters by becoming a surrogate mother. They may as well have been talking to themselves, though, for Jane had made up her mind. She was going to be a surrogate mother.

"It was fate; it was destiny. I couldn't fight it. At least this was what she told herself whenever her practical side began to impress her with reminders that surrogacy wasn't a known, well-tested or even simple procedure. Even at the height of her romantic musings about bearing someone else's child, Jane knew that this was still essentially uncharted territory. This was made quite clear to her on a visit to an attorney regarding the contract between herself, the clinic, and the couple. The lawyer had grave misgivings about surrogacy. He told Jane that surrogate parenting was not recognized in Massachusetts courts. Under those circumstances, he feared that Jane would lose out if the other parties involved did not uphold their end of the contract.

By this time Jane was so determined to become a surrogate mother that it would have taken all the powers of the universe to talk her out of it. She rationalized that the money would help her family; it would give her more time with her two little girls. In private moments she admitted that she needed to do this for a more personal reason: she had to create life again, even if it meant relinquishing that life to the care of someone else. So Jane didn't follow her attorney's advice to give up on surrogacy. But neither was she altogether starry-eyed about the prospect. She knew better than to sign away the use of her body without ensuring that some provisions were included in the contract to protect herself and her family. For example, she asked for and received a contractual change to include payment of child care while she was hospitalized. (The couple was bound by contract to pay all medical expenses related to the pregnancy, the birth, and any medical difficulties ensuing from the birth.) She also refused to sign on as a surrogate mother unless the couple agreed to pay for any alternative medical care she desired.

The couple complied with her requests, the contracts were signed, and the next issue was when she would be inseminated. Because of the move and her new job, Jane requested that this be postponed until August. All parties agreed, and she began to keep track of her fertility pattern. Her earlier feelings of trepidation vanished, and Jane felt only "excitement" at the prospect of carrying and bearing this new life.

One day in August around the time of ovulation, Jane took her temperature and determined that she was fertile. She called Elaine immediately and then headed for the clinic for the insemination process. The insemination took place in a doctor's office down the hall from Elaine's small suite. Jane remembers being ushered into the office and taken to an examining room. Meanwhile, the prospective father was in the clinic office producing a semen specimen. This was carried to the doctor's office where the gynecologist on call examined it under the microscope to determine whether the sperm were alive and active. They were. He placed the sample in a small syringe without a needle. When he entered the examining room Jane, already undressed, lay on the examining table. She remembers the doctor telling her that the sperm were very active before he inserted the syringe into her vagina. The insemination process lasted only seconds. When the doctor withdrew the syringe, Jane was told she should wait on the table for twenty minutes with her hips elevated in order to facilitate the fertilization process. Two days later she underwent a second insemination at the same doctor's office as a backup measure.

There was never any doubt in Jane's mind that she had been impregnated by the first insemination. In the interim, before her next period was due, she took a vacation with her children to Block Island. Although they stayed with close friends, she didn't mention her possible physical condition to anyone. She tried to enjoy the scenery and the company of people, but her thoughts were lost in the changes she sensed were taking place inside her.

As Jane had expected, she missed her next period, and the blood test came back positive. She was pregnant, and ecstatic about it. "Even though I was sick, I felt gleeful," she said. Given the circumstances of her pregnancy, Jane told no one until the first trimester had passed and she had had an amniocentesis to check on the health of the fetus. She learned that she was carrying a healthy baby girl. The amniocentesis was not a process Jane would have chosen for herself, but she went along to please the couple. After all she was over 35, and the chances of a birth defect increase with the age of the mother.

As soon as her pregnancy was confirmed, Jane began to prepare her daughters for the impending birth. "I took them on my bed and I told them about infertility," she said. "I told them that I was having a baby for another family who had a little girl. I explained that they needed another little girl so they could be like us. I explained how the scientists had put in the seed to grow in my body. They were very accepting. Children don't have preconceived notions of morality. My older daughter wanted to keep the baby, or for me to have another, but I told her that we couldn't afford it."

Once the worry about the children was out of the way,

Jane said she coped well with the early stages of her pregnancy. Still, she found herself feeling increasingly exhausted with the effort of supporting her family. After a bout with the flu, which left her drained, she left her job as a pool nurse at the local hospital and took a less desirable position in a nursing home where the hours were more convenient.

The new job served a dual purpose. Because Jane was a stranger at the nursing home, she didn't have to discuss her background or surrogacy. Knowing that she wouldn't start showing until midwinter, she kept quiet about the pregnancy. It was a secret: "The neighbors didn't know until spring. My coworkers thought I had a husband." She didn't tell her parents until Christmas, and then only because she and the girls were visiting them. "It was very hard for them to take," she recalled. "They said to me, 'Why don't you just be normal? You have enough stresses in your life. Why take on another?' "

The visit to her parents' home was probably the most uncomfortable experience of Jane's pregnancy—apart from problems she had with a boyfriend and her former husband. She said her parents were ill at ease around her and a little ashamed: "They didn't want anyone to know. I told them I was doing this because I wanted to do it. I didn't tell them the complicated reasons. At least my two brothers thought it was fine."

If her parents were uncomfortable about her plans, Jane's former husband was so hostile that he threatened to sue her for custody of their two girls. Terrified of this prospect, Jane suggested that they go into counseling over the issue. He reluctantly agreed for the children's sake. What the counseling revealed was that he was angry because the baby wasn't his.

Eventually he agreed to drop all talk of a custody suit. As the pregnancy drew to a close, the man Jane had been dating dropped out of her life. He couldn't deal with the pregnancy either. Also traumatic for Jane was coping with the expected inquiries from well-meaning people about the sex of the baby and when it was due. She found herself lying about her situation to avoid discussing the surrogacy with strangers. Although she understood their curiosity, she was frequently annoyed when people touched her stomach. It was even more difficult when her little girls blurted out information about the pregnancy that she would have preferred to have kept private. From time to time they informed strangers that "Mommy's giving her baby away," to the general disquiet of everyone involved. Despite these disturbances Jane said she enjoyed this pregnancy as she had her others. She liked the way pregnancy forced her to "think more internally" and only regretted that she had little leisure in which to enjoy this meditative state. During the entire process she said she never felt alone or lacked support the way she had with her first two pregnancies. What kept her going during those months before she was due—was a nourishing sense of being part of this new life she had created to give away.

In the early hours of April 29 Jane's waters broke while she was sleeping. She emerged from a dream not quite certain what had happened, then became frightened that she might have a repeat of her first pregnancy during which labor had been induced. If labor does not start on its own within twelve hours of the waters breaking, most doctors will induce it to protect the fetus. Jane knew she was safe from that fate when she felt the first contraction at about 2:00 P.M. that day. It was very mild, and was followed by a second contraction ten minutes later. This, too, was quite mild. At 2:30 P.M. she called the midwife. Convinced that delivery was hours away, Jane calmly took care of the arrangements she had made for her daughters before calling her labor coach. By 3:00 P.M. there had been several contractions in quick succession. The midwife instructed her to get to the hospital right away. No sooner had Jane hung up the phone than the contractions began coming three minutes apart. Her friend, who was doubling as labor coach, picked her up in a big van. As they drove along the tree-lined streets of the town, Jane clutched her stomach and was grateful that she wasn't driving herself the eight blocks to the small red-brick country hospital.

If the ride seemed endless, Jane described the admitting process as being "painfully slow." The baby was ready to arrive and they were making her fill out form after form. Birth was so imminent, that Jane feared she would have the baby in the middle of the cramped admitting office. As the clerk typed in her vital statistics, she contemplated marching off to the birthing room without the necessary forms.

At last she was officially admitted. Feeling as if the baby was about to "fall out," Jane quickly made her way to the birthing room off the maternity ward. Friends—her nursing colleagues—smiled as she settled into what looked like a motel room done up in burnt orange. But there was little time to contemplate her surroundings or even to answer routine questions. "The baby's coming soon," she told a nurse who had stopped by to take her blood pressure, temperature, and medical history. Already, Jane was lying on her side breathing through the contractions. As with her other two children, she had a "back labor," which means that the fetus was facing toward the back causing stress in that region. But even though this baby had caught her off guard with the speed of its arrival, Jane felt prepared and in control. Concentrating on the contractions, she tried to keep her mind above the pain.

Her main disappointment was that her older daughter, the five-year-old, couldn't be there to witness the birth of her half sister. The little girl had begged to be allowed to come, and Jane had acceded, but not before sending her to a special children's class on childbirth. After all that preparation, labor had begun while her daughter was in school. Irrational as it later seemed to Jane, while she lay in the hospital about to give birth, she felt as if she had cheated her daughter of an experience by giving birth during school hours.

Then events came together so fast that she had no time to think about her daughter or the people who would take this baby from her within twenty-four hours after its birth. Neither was there time to think about whether she regretted going through all this pain for the sake of an infertile couple and $10,000. She was concentrating all her energies on pushing the baby out of her body. What she wanted was as natural a childbirth as possible—a birth without unnecessary drugs or cutting. She was determined to stay in control of the situation.

The baby was born at 4:19 P.M., half an hour after Jane's arrival at the hospital. This birth was very different from her first two. There had been minimal tearing, and Jane felt she had been in control the entire time. "This time I knew what was happening, she said. "I was completely aware. I felt my mission was accomplished on that level. I was elated, on cloud nine. I couldn't come down." The baby had emerged slightly blue and was immediately administered oxygen. As the child was not hers to keep, Jane decided to allow her whatever conventional medical treatment the doctors recommended. She did not feel she should impose her own medical philosophy on others. She herself refused drugs to stop the uterine bleeding that commonly follows birth.

Jane asked for the infant almost as soon as she was out of the womb. She lay the tiny, 7.4-pound creature on her stomach and pushed her breast to its mouth. The baby started sucking, releasing the contracting agents in Jane's body. The uterine bleeding soon stopped. One of Jane's stipulations before agreeing to be a surrogate mother was that she be allowed to nurse the baby while the two of them were together in the hospital. The other request was that the baby remain with her in the birthing room except when Jane was sleeping. Jane wanted to feel a connection with the infant before giving her up forever.

As the baby sucked at her breast, Jane surveyed the little body that had been a part of her for nine months. The baby had darkish hair, and from the nose down she resembled Jane's two daughters. "Her eyes," Jane reflected, "were her father's." Even though she was giving up this infant, at that moment Jane thought of her as her baby. I felt "so proud to have produced such a beautiful and healthy baby," she said, looking back. "I felt waves of love, but not attachment. A girlfriend has said to me that only I could do this. Maybe that's because I think of love more as giving than as keeping, though I would never give away my own children. But this was the father's child."

The private moment between surrogate mother and child was cut short by the arrival of the clinic director. Excited and thrilled at the birth, Elaine was soon on the phone to the expectant couple. Before Jane could comprehend what had happened, Elaine was handing her the phone. Jane remembers the woman offering her congratulations. She replied, "No, it's congratulations to you." That call was hardly out of the way before the baby-sitter brought up Jane's daughters. The five-year-old glanced at the baby and then spent the rest of the visit playing on the floor with her toys. The three-year-old, on the other hand, wanted to hold the infant and barraged Jane with questions.

The little girls had no sooner gone home than Elaine came in to tell Jane that the adoptive parents had arrived. She wheeled out the baby in its bassinet. Jane said she experienced no sense of loss at the time, only excitement at the thought that the parents were going to be seeing the baby for the first time. "I wanted to be a fly on the wall of the room they were in so I could see their reaction," she said. If she experienced any sadness, Jane hardly had a chance to contemplate it. Not long after Elaine had taken the baby out, one of Jane's brothers stopped by with champagne and strawberries for a celebration. About twenty minutes later, Elaine returned with the surprising news that the couple wanted to meet Jane. Was she willing?

"Of course, I said yes," Jane reported. "I preferred contact with the parents. It made me feel part of something." Until that moment, though she wasn't certain she would ever meet the baby's parents. Prior to the birth, she had been undecided whether a face-to-face visit was a good idea. The other woman had been adamantly opposed to it. But when Elaine presented her with this option in the birthing room of the hospital, Jane knew that she did indeed want to meet the people who would raise this baby—her biological baby.

Jane had very little inkling of what to expect. Her only previous view of the couple was a ten-year-old picture. What she saw when they walked through the door were two extremely happy people. Two "vital, fit, casual, warm people." She liked them. She liked their unpretentiousness, their kindness, and their "homey, parental look." The meeting didn't last long. The couple left, the baby was removed to the nursery so Jane could sleep, and for the first time since her waters broke early that morning she was alone in this room that made her feel as if she was in a motel. She wished she were in her comfy brown bungalow filled with kids and kids' things. For a long time Jane was unable to sleep. It wasn't that she was filled with doubts about what she had done. She needed time to mentally process the events of the day—and there had been so many events. Meeting the parents, for example, had left her feeling strangely relieved. She realized after they left that she would have felt "bereft" if she hadn't met them. The meeting had served as a resolution of the surrogate parenting period. And then there was the baby and the elation she had felt at the success of the birth. "I had this funny sense of contentedness that things had come to pass. It was like something out of the Bible," Jane said. "There was no sense of anything gone awry. Things had gone better than I thought they would."

Once during the night the baby was brought in for nursing. She was back in the birthing room with Jane the next morning when the parents arrived and told the staff they wanted to take the baby home. The doctors said the baby was slightly jaundiced and they needed to do some blood tests first. That was about 10:00 A.M. The couple could have gone elsewhere during the delay, but they chose to stay with Jane until they received word that the baby could be released. They ended up spending two hours together. The talk centered around the logistics of how Jane would get breast milk to them. They exchanged phone numbers. Slowly, as things began to feel more comfortable, more personal items crept into the conversation. The couple talked about their six-year-old daughter—their natural child—and about their childbearing attitudes. Jane liked the fact that they didn't seem pushy or overly achievement oriented. "They seemed in tune with their child's needs. Family was important. So was culture," she concluded.

The fact that these people seemed deeply caring also made things easier for Jane. She realized that she couldn't have been a surrogate for just anyone. She couldn't have gone through all this unless she felt some psychic connection. And with these people she had felt that connection from the time Elaine had first mentioned their names—a feeling that grew on her as they corresponded during the pregnancy. Meeting them helped to confirm the psychic connection. They were different from many surrogate parenting couples in that there was always the possibility they might conceive again. In fact, Jane believed they were still trying to have another child by natural means. She told them she prayed they could have another baby. "I don't want to keep having babies for you," she half joked.

For Jane the parents' obvious delight with the baby made everything feel right. "The baby was conceived as a gift," she said. "I was able to see that completion. I think it would be harder for other people. I knew she was mine for nine months. Then she would be the parents' for twenty years and her own person for the rest of her life. I had the privilege of having that first nine months. I don't have to go through the diaper period, the staying up with a sick child, or the teenage years—none of the difficulties of parenthood. Yet I got to know her intimately. I did my parenting stint with her." These thoughts got Jane through many difficult moments during her stint as surrogate mother, beginning with the pregnancy and birth and ending with the hospitalization and final good-byes to the baby. When the couple left her bedside, there was no talk of future contact outside of Jane's providing the baby with breast milk. She readily signed the baby over to them as stipulated in the contract and left things at that. If that action caused her pain, Jane didn't acknowledge it then. The baby was the couple's to keep.

Jane returned home to her two little girls twenty-four hours after giving birth. Within days she had resumed her old routine of working, cooking, grocery shopping, and caring for the children. For the first two weeks after labor she said she felt fine emotionally but was extremely tired. The fact that her children seemed to need her more increased her exhaustion. Both were upset to find that no baby had accompanied Mommy home. There was little Jane could do except pray that this experience would not leave any psychological wounds. And so things went until three weeks after the birth when she received a notice from the couple's lawyer. In formal, legal terminology it announced that she had "forever" relinquished her rights as mother of this child. Jane was shaken by the letter. Nothing had felt real until she received that letter. She had to sit for a while and absorb the shock of the realization that "this was final. It couldn't be revoked."

As the weeks passed, Jane found herself swinging between wishing she could maintain contact with the baby— even as a kind of aunt—and feeling that it was best that they were separate. For a while she wanted to know about her: what she was doing, how much she weighed, whether she was smiling. She longed for a picture the parents had promised to send her. As spring turned to summer, though, her interest slackened. By mid-June she had stopped supplying breast milk and no longer wished for contact with the baby and her parents. As she distanced herself emotionally she found that she still wanted to know the baby but not to have her: "I recognized that that wasn't my right," she said. "But I suspected from time to time I would want her to know about me."

There was also the issue of the $10,000 Jane earned for her services as a surrogate mother. The couple had paid her while she was in the hospital, but at first Jane couldn't bring herself to cash the check. "I felt upset about the material aspect of this," she said. "It took me two weeks to deposit it." After six weeks she still hadn't touched the money. At the sight of her many unpaid bills, though, Jane found herself reaching into the fund. Freed of her self-imposed taboo about spending her earnings, she decided to use the remaining funds to put her little girls into private school. She would provide them with private schooling as long as the money lasted.

With the spending came the realization that $10,000 really doesn't go very far. "It isn't really much," Jane admitted. "Some people tell me it wasn't enough, considering what I did. They're right. It isn't enough. But how do you put a value on what I've done?" Jane has no answers except to go on with her life. In early summer she began a new job as a maternity-ward nurse at a hospital in a neighboring state. She loves the job, the hours, and the fact that she works in a birthing center where the attitudes are liberal and holistic medicine is practiced. She's also studying to be a teacher of the Lamaze childbirth method.

As the first anniversary of the insemination drew near, Jane felt a semblance of normalcy settling over her life. She and her boyfriend have had a reconciliation even though it hasn't been a conflict-free relationship. He has children from a previous marriage and has told Jane that he doesn't want any more. To continue with this man might mean an end to her childbearing hopes. But because Jane is undecided about having future children herself, she has decided to stay with the relationship. If she's learned anything in recent years, it's that "you don't compromise yourself to have kids."

Looking back on her experience as a surrogate mother, Jane can see that the reality proved to be very different from her fantasies. She thought she would have an opportunity to relive her first two births. She thought she would be able to keep a diary or journal during the course of the pregnancy and use her experiences as material for a thesis, but there was no time to write down anything. Now her memory of minute details has faded. All the same, she feels that interesting things have emerged from this act of bearing life for others: "It's been a birth and rebirth for me. I look at it as my birth, not the baby's. Things in life seem to be opening up. Years of turmoil and suffering are dissolving, and I feel I'm finally evolving freer and with more power. I attribute that to the pregnancy. When you're creating life, you're making a spiritual force material. As a result, I found something more spiritual in me. Then I released it."

This will probably be the last time Jane seeks a spiritual release in quite this fashion. For the most part she's decided against a repeat performance as a surrogate mother. Her daughters are the main reason. She doesn't want to send them the message that you use your body for money. The one-time experience was healthy, she said, because it taught the girls something about giving to others and was "a good experience in human sexuality."

As much as Jane's life has fallen into place, though, there are still times when she has emotional twinges. For instance, she gets teary-eyed when she sees little babies with their mothers. And she was deeply saddened when the friend who served as her labor coach subsequently lost her own baby through a miscarriage. Then there are the awkward moments when people ask her about the baby. Jane simply tells them she's with her father. There are also times when she wants to confide in people about the baby, but she feels they won't understand. Often she's right. For the few who say "That's wonderful," there are many more who tell her, "You couldn't pay me to do that."

Although Jane recognizes that it's difficult for others to understand, she feels good about what she's done. She looks upon the birth of this child she may never know as an accomplishment. "I achieved a goal," she said. Yet because of public opinion, Jane's act remains primarily a private one, and the child she bore her personal tribute to life and the miracle of birth. "I have the sense that someday we will meet again in an unattached way," she said. "I won't make that happen; she'll have to. It may not happen and that's okay." Clearly, Jane carries her scars. But she insists there are no regrets.

# 6 | Surrogate Mothers: A National Survey

When Mary Beth Whitehead refused to give up "Baby M" to the New Jersey couple who had contracted for the child's birth, the nation's media initiated a campaign to determine what sort of woman becomes a surrogate mother. Scouring the country, journalists found a variety of psychologists who were willing to describe the average surrogate mother; and while they came up with a profile of sorts, it was generally admitted that there is a lack of hard data on the subject.

Ms. Surrogate Mother was said to be white, Christian and in her thirties, with at least a high school education and one child of her own. If the demographics seemed a little sketchy, it was because at the time of the Stern-Whitehead trial no comprehensive, nationwide study of surrogate mothers had yet been conducted. The research that had been done involved limited samples and concentrated on defining what motivates a woman to act as a surrogate mother. From these studies—a smattering of which emerged in media interviews with professionals in the sur-

rogate parenting field during the course of the "Baby M" trial—came the general conclusion that money isn't the major
motivating factor that drives women to have babies for others. Altruism, a need to feel good about themselves or make
a special contribution to society, guilt over past abortions,
personal experiences as adoptive children, the need to reen-
act their own childhood abandonment, and other deep psychological factors were found to be the primary reasons
women agree to act as surrogate mothers.

One of those experts whose work received much attention was Philip J. Parker, the Michigan psychiatrist who
screens surrogates for Noel Keane's surrogate parenting
program—the program that matched the Whiteheads and
the Sterns. Parker had conducted a study of 125 surrogates
in 1983 in which it was revealed that money, a desire to be
pregnant, and an interest in reconciling past birth-related
traumas were the three main reasons women chose to be
surrogate mothers. He also concluded, however, that altruism was not as great a motivating factor as some surrogates
insist. In later studies involving a sampling of 500 surrogates, Parker reportedly found that at least one-third of the
women had gone through an abortion or given up a baby for
adoption. Another 10 percent, according to Parker, were
themselves adopted children and participated in the surrogacy program as a way of expressing gratitude to their adoptive parents.

Because of his connection with Keane and the "Baby M"
case, Parker's data and his screening techniques for Keane's
clinic came under close scrutiny during the course of the
custody battle. Of special interest was the fact that Parker
rarely rejects a prospective candidate for surrogacy but ap-
proves any woman who understands the ramifications of
her actions. According to Parker there is no way "to predict
with any certainty how a surrogate mother will do psychologically, or whether she will decide to keep the child." Giv-
en the lack of conclusive data, he believes the question of

whether to disqualify a woman from a surrogate parenting program is, "for the time being a moral question, not a scientific one." Isadore Schmukler, a clinical psychologist who screens surrogates applying to the Surrogate Mother Program in New York City, subscribes to the theory that most surrogates are motivated by the need to do something very special. He contends that most surrogates see themselves "as able to give an extraordinary gift to a couple in need."

Although Parker's and Schmukler's psychological assessments may well be on target, something is lacking in these and similar studies that appeared in the media throughout the period in which the "Baby M" case was headline news. That "something" was a sense of surrogate mothers as living, breathing human beings—diverse human beings, at that. For after talking with Jane Woodman and a number of other surrogates about their personal experiences, it became evident to me that there is no single stereotype that describes all surrogate mothers. The survey taken for this book confirmed that many were white, Christian, single parents in their thirties; but there were many who could not be so neatly pigeonholed. Many worked in the nurturing end of the medical professions—nursing was well represented— and many did not. the only thing all surrogate mothers seemed to have in common was their surrogacy. A look at the case histories of three former surrogate mothers revealed three very different women with three very different personalities acting on three very different sets of priorities.

Kate, a twenty-one-year-old native New Englander who lives in North Carolina, turned to surrogacy to lift herself out of poverty. At the age of seventeen, she had become pregnant and had given up her baby girl to foster care. Devastated by the experience and very broke, she responded to an advertisement for surrogate mothers. Despite her own rocky childhood—she was a product of foster homes—and young age, she was accepted into a surrogate parenting program. She became pregnant easily and lived through a very lonely nine-month pregnancy during which she felt the couple involved neglected and mistreated her. "They felt I was a nineteen-year-old punk doing it for the money," she recalled.

In fact, Kate has admitted that money was a large motivating factor in her decision to become a surrogate mother. With the fee from the first pregnancy and a second stint as a surrogate mother—a more positive experience this time—she was able to purchase a mobile home and bring her three-year-old daughter home. For Kate, who had not yet been reunited with her little girl, the second surrogate birth was agony. She learned during the pregnancy that she was bearing a girl and often contemplated keeping the baby. Only loyalty to the couple she was working with made her stick to the agreement. In retrospect, she said she would relive her surrogacy experiences all over again if the money she could earn from surrogacy would help "bring consistency into my three-year-old's life." But with a steady job as a day-care worker and a child to raise, Kate stated pointedly that she would not act as a surrogate mother a third time.

Laurie Johnson is about as far from the stereotypical image of a surrogate mother as you can get. A video producer who formerly wrote for television and was involved in the Detroit, Michigan, area theater, this strong, assertive woman said she went into surrogate parenting for "selfish" reasons. She wanted to experience pregnancy without "getting emotionally involved in a baby." Not that Laurie dislikes children or wouldn't want a child of her own. But as a divorcee in her thirties with no marital prospects in sight, she felt she couldn't pass up the opportunity to live through a pregnancy. Although there were difficult moments during the surrogacy experience, moments when she wished for emotional support, Laurie said she suffered no recrimination from friends or family.

Her work situation was a different story. The winter following the birth she was fired from her job, ostensibly on the grounds of poor work performance. Laurie believes her involvement in surrogate parenting was the real cause. Despite this experience, she has no regrets about being a surrogate mother. Following the "Baby M" case, Laurie began actively lobbying nationwide on behalf of the procedure. She also plans to bear a second child for her couple, whom she now regards as friends. About surrogacy Laurie said: "I was able to have a really great experience without paying for it. Taking care of a child isn't in the cards for me without a husband. But this has been the perfect situation. Still, it's important to note that I know myself."

Then there's Jan Sutton, who, as spokeswoman of the National Association of Surrogate Mothers, has been working hard to gain respect for women like herself. A San Diego nurse in her late thirties and the divorced mother of two, Jan served twice as a surrogate mother for the Los Angeles—based Center of Surrogate Parenting—the same center that spawned the National Association of Surrogate Mothers. Jan's interest in surrogacy was sparked by personal knowledge of the "heartache infertility can bring." Of the four children in her family, only she and one other child were her parents' natural children. "I knew my parents had wanted more children and couldn't have them. I knew how extremely unhappy they were," she reported.

Although she has had no infertility problems of her own, Jan experienced some of her parents' anguish when her husband had a vasectomy after their two children were born. Feeling that two children were enough, she had agreed to the operation. Afterward, she found it hard to accept that her childbearing years were over. Then, in 1983, a television show on surrogate parenting caught her eye and she knew she had to do something: "I know it might sound selfish, but I wanted to be pregnant again. I just didn't want to take the child home." After mulling over her decision for several months she found the telephone number of the Center of Surrogate Parenting and applied to their program. Because of the distance between San Diego and Los Angeles, Jan was uncertain whether she would be accepted. To her surprise she was. "They accepted me," she said, "because I looked like a very stable person who had examined what she was doing. I was also a professional who had dealt with children. They felt I would do very well as a surrogate mother. I was the sort of person a couple would want."

Although Jan didn't know it then, she would end up acting as a surrogate mother twice. She met her first couple at the end of 1983, and the child was born the following October. The center introduced her to a second couple in the winter of 1984, and the baby was born in December of that year. For Jan, money had very little to do with her involvement in surrogacy. If anything, she considers the money she received for her two stints as a surrogate mother as recompense for hard work. Looking back at all her expenses— travel costs, hotel rooms—and all the time spent away from family members, any suggestion that she did this for the money irritates her. She insists that her compensation was witnessing the joy on the faces of the couples she made happy. "I still get goose pimples remembering the faces of my first couple in the delivery room. It was sitting there in the delivery room that I made the decision to do it again. It was an extremely worthwhile experience. It was beautiful."

Beautiful as it was, Jan felt that serving twice as a surrogate mother was enough. She and her husband were divorced after the second pregnancy for reasons unrelated to her surrogacy, and she did not want to go through another pregnancy as a single parent. "Anyway," she said, "I felt that twice was enough. Someone else would worry that I was becoming a breeder; I just felt satisfied. I'd accomplished what I wanted. I'd made two couples a family, and that made me extremely happy." Rather than remove herself from the field, Jan has continued her involvement in surrogate parenting in another way. Because of her outgoing nature she found herself, in the fall of 1986 acting as spokeswoman of the newly formed National Association of Surrogate Mothers. Now her main objective is to educate people about surrogate parenting and to let them know that it's a "fabulous" experience. "We have several goals," she said. "One is to get positive media coverage about surrogate parenting. We want to maintain it as a viable option for couples. And we want guidelines set up for clinics so not just anyone can hang up a shingle. We realize that the surrogate needs support throughout the process and the family needs support."

Most of the twenty-five surrogate mothers interviewed for this book echoed Jan's sentiments. Many are single mothers working in nurturing fields such as health care or early childhood education. About half of them lived in California; the rest came from Connecticut, Iowa, Kansas, Massachusetts, Michigan, Missouri, North Carolina, and Washington State. All told, between 20,000 and 25,000 women contacted surrogate parenting programs between 1980 and 1987 to inquire about becoming surrogate mothers. About 4,300 made inquiries in 1986 alone, with about half of these accepted into one program or another. Clinic directors reportedly accept twice the number of surrogates as couples in order to ensure availability.

Although the women in the informal sample interviewed for this book came from different parts of the country and represented a variety of cultural and educational backgrounds, they were very much united by their shared experience of surrogacy and by their enjoyment of the process. Most of them cannot understand a world that looks askance at bearing a child for others. Most of them felt that they have contributed to society by their actions, and more than half of them have said they would do it again.

All the surrogates interviewed were involved with surrogate parenting clinics or centers. Compared with the couples surveyed, the surrogates evinced a marked attitudinal difference between those involved with West Coast clinics and those who worked with clinics located elsewhere. This may be because clinics on the West Coast—especially in California—stress contact with the couple far more than do clinics in other parts of the country. Consequently, the relationship with the couple appears to have been far more important to West Coast surrogates than to their counterparts in Massachusetts or Kansas, for example.

Most of the women in this sample expressed more than one reason for becoming a surrogate. Even so, almost all of them placed altruism—or doing something for others—at the top of their list. Next was their enjoyment of being pregnant, followed by their desire to do something that gave them a feeling of pride. Only two of the women interviewed mentioned money; and one surrogate said she wanted to experience pregnancy with her second husband without the burden of childbearing. There were surrogates—largely from California—who said they offered their services to infertile couples because they "saw a need for it." Like Jan, many of these surrogate mothers had had personal experiences with infertility or had close friends or relatives who suffered from their inability to have children.

A surrogate mother from Connecticut said she was first moved to help at the age of eighteen when she befriended an infertile woman. Her chance came years later when she saw a television special on surrogate parenting, tracked down a clinic in a nearby state, and offered her services. Looking back over her experience, she realized that she did this "out of wanting to help someone." A surrogate mother from another New England State reported that "to do something in my lifetime that you don't always get a chance to do and pay some bills" was her motive for becoming involved in surrogate parenting. And for a surrogate from Massachusetts, getting involved was originally done "100 percent for the money". "But," she continued, "as time went on I realized how many people were unable to have children of their own. I felt very proud that I would be able to give to someone a child that was really wanted and would be loved and cared for probably more than half of the children brought into this world."

In January 1987, during the course of the "Baby M" trial, a number of surrogate mothers granted interviews to *Newsweek*. These women generally reflected what psychologists and clinic directors had learned—that women often turn to surrogacy as a means of giving. And for them, giving is a form of personal expression. Becky McKnight, a Los Angeles mother of three, told *Newsweek* (Jan. 19, 1987) that she became a surrogate after seeing "the disappointment and the anguish that accompanies infertility." In the same article Carolyn Williams, a San Francisco surrogate, said she regarded surrogacy as a personal calling: "I feel that God gave me this gift. I left the hospital with a picture in my mind of happiness—a happy family." And Lisa Walters, a Grantsburg, Wisconsin, surrogate, said she couldn't cure cancer or become Mother Teresa, "but a baby is one thing I can sort of give back; something I can give to someone else who couldn't have it any other way."

A surprisingly large percentage of women who chose surrogacy for the first time—half of those surveyed—found that the process was in keeping with their own high ideals. These women tended to bring to this new experience the generally rosy assessment of pregnancy and motherhood usually associated with a first birth despite the fact that most of them already had children of their own. Of course, most of these women also loved being pregnant and reported having easy deliveries. Interestingly, none of the surrogates reported having any initial qualms about the procedure, and about one-fifth of them claimed to have had no expectations whatever. California surrogates reported having expectations not expressed by surrogates in other parts of the country when it came to forming relationships with their couple and making them happy. These women also tended to put more emphasis on self-fulfillment. In general, the West

Coast surrogates seemed more confident about the process and the outcome. Perhaps because attendance in support groups is mandatory at a number of California surrogate parenting centers, these surrogates appear to have been better able to anticipate the pitfalls of surrogate motherhood while enjoying what they considered to be the joyous aspects of the experience.

While one-third of the nationwide sample found the physical aspects of surrogacy to be better than they had anticipated, most California surrogates found that their pregnancies and deliveries proceeded pretty much as they had expected. California surrogates expected their experience to be positive as a matter of course. As for the emotional aspect, one-third of the sample found the procedure to be better than anticipated as compared with one-fifth of those from California.

Nationally, surrogates who reported negative experiences were in a distinct minority. Among those who did have problems, the most common complaints noted were a feeling of letdown following the birth, lack of support from physicians, harried clinics, and uncaring couples. At times, too, these women reported having to cope with hypercritical friends, relatives, and coworkers. Some lost jobs, boyfriends, or had sexual complications as a result of the insemination. Others reported being plagued by their fears of creating an imperfect child. While they shared many of these concerns, California surrogates had their own set of complaints. Several women were upset at finding that there was less involvement with their couples than they had anticipated. Others were dismayed at the amount of waiting they were forced to endure before actually conceiving. And a few reported being accidentally impregnated by their husbands.

When they were asked to comment on what they found to be the most positive aspect of their surrogacy experience, an overwhelming number of surrogates reported that the end result was very much what they had hoped for—pure joy at having done something special for someone else. Just under one-third of the sample found that they loved being pregnant—as they had predicted—and a similar number reported that surrogacy enhanced their personal development. One-fifth of those surveyed said that, along with other aspects of surrogacy, the money was an added benefit that made the experience worthwhile. A number of California surrogates also reported enjoying the social benefits of belonging to a support group.

Discussing her experience, one surrogate mother on the East Coast—who was thrilled with the outcome but disgruntled with the process—said she would have liked more support before and after the baby was born. In her case, neither the clinic nor the doctor was particularly caring. The doctor was downright nasty, she felt, and went so far as to refuse to deliver the baby, while the clinic director was preoccupied. Although the doctor was prevailed upon to deliver the baby the surrogate said he was surly and insulting. This kind of horror story among surrogate mothers was rare. Most of the women interviewed for this book discovered that their minor fears and concerns did not mar the overall experience. Jan Sutton, for example, worried about producing an imperfect child for her first couple. After sitting down and talking with them about her fears, however, she realized that they were groundless.

Surrogates who reported having difficult pregnancies and deliveries found that support from the clinic and the couple made all the difference. Said one surrogate, "I had a lot of support from everyone involved and we made it through. It was one of the best feelings in my life to see how happy these people were about their new child." Other surrogate mothers found that a loving, caring spouse or friend could be an invaluable asset. Lisa Walters told *Newsweek* that when she ignited a family feud with her decision to become a surrogate—her inlaws reportedly threatened to take her and her husband to court and remove their children from the household on grounds that she was an unfit mother—her husband sided with her and as a result their marriage improved. Eight months pregnant at the time of the interview, she said she had no regrets about her actions.

People who look at surrogacy from the outside assume that giving up the baby is the hardest aspect of serving as a surrogate mother. This was found to be true for only one-fifth of the women interviewed for this book. More than half of those surveyed said they were well prepared for relinquishment. In fact, most of these surrogates never considered the baby to be theirs in the first place. New York clinical psychologist Isadore Schmukler believes that surrogates are able to cushion themselves against the pain of giving up their babies. He has not seen much fantasizing about the baby among the surrogates he has screened for the Surrogate Mother Program in New York. "From the beginning they lack the usual emotional tie. They don't perceive it psychologically as theirs," he observed.

"It is never difficult to give away what is not yours to begin with," said a surrogate mother from Iowa. "Life is a gift from God. He helped to create this life especially for the parents, not for me. It's a little bit like the time I designed and created a dress for my sister to wear to the prom. It was my creation, but Sis paid for the materials. I enjoyed making the dress. I was proud of my creation, but I didn't want to keep it for myself." Another surrogate said she found giving up the baby easier than she had originally expected because she "knew it was their baby from the beginning. Being well prepared made it easier to give up the baby. Also," she added, "it looked like the father." A surrogate who had already been through the sleepless nights and diaper stage with her own two children said she had "no desire to deal with that business again! Some people," she continued, "ask me if I ever think about the baby. Of course I do. But I know that the baby will have everything it will ever need."

In her work with The National Association of Surrogate

Mothers, Jan Sutton said she has never met a surrogate who wanted to keep the baby or make life difficult for the couple. "Surrogates would never do that to a couple because it's the father's child more than theirs," she said. According to Jan, saying good-bye to the couple can be the hardest thing a surrogate mother has to do. "They think of them as friends. Some of these are true friendships with deep bonds." Surrogates who found it difficult to relinquish the child, it was found, had usually given birth to a child of a sex they had wanted but had not produced for their own families. Jan has also found that surrogates who had previously given up babies for adoption were more likely to find relinquishment emotionally trying. One surrogate mother had two boys by her husband but had privately always wanted a girl. When she gave birth to a baby girl as part of a surrogate parenting program she felt she was "giving up the one thing I wanted most all my life. It was very difficult. I coped with the pain by burying it."

Most of the surrogate mothers interviewed for this book felt that it was easier to give up the child once they had established contact with the couple. The majority of surrogate mothers interviewed met their couple before proceeding with the insemination. Some, like Laurie Johnson, have developed a lasting friendship; others stay in touch on a first-name basis only; and some met once at the hospital and will probably never see one another again. All of the mothers who have maintained contact reported being glad they did so. However, they have acknowledged that creating temporary relationships can also mean creating painful breakups. Several California surrogates have found breaking contact with their couple to be more difficult than giving up the child. "What works for some doesn't work for others," Jan Sutton said of anonymity. "I know cases where letters and phone calls can work. Personally, I couldn't have done it without contact. I had to meet the people to build trust. You can't build a relationship of trust with an inanimate object."

Although a few surrogates who have maintained strict anonymity have admitted a preference for operating that way, others wish they had met their couple. Or at the very least, they would have liked to have known more about them. "They know everything about us and we know nothing about them," was a common complaint. "I feel like I've given up a baby to strangers," one surrogate lamented. Another surrogate, who finally met her couple in the hospital after the birth, said she felt heartened by the contact. "If everything had gone smoothly, I wanted them in the delivery room. But we never got that far due to complications in my pregnancy. They came to visit me a few times in the hospital and, yes, I'm glad they did. The joy these people had gave me such a good feeling. I have not one regret for having met them."

Bearing a child for other people may be wonderful, but accepting money for that service is quite another issue. Given their altruistic leanings, most surrogates—even those who were supportive of the fees they received—appeared to be somewhat uncomfortable about the money their services garnered. While three-quarters of those interviewed supported receiving payment, they were careful to identify the fee as remuneration—very much a necessary evil—for their efforts rather than as payment for a baby.

Despite general acceptance of the necessity of some financial compensation, feelings about payment varied widely among surrogates. One-third of them reported feeling ambivalent about accepting money for what they had done. A handful said they did not feel they had been paid sufficiently for their services. However, none of the women felt they would have become a surrogate mother if they had not been offered financial compensation for their time and efforts. According to one surrogate, the $10,000 fee was fine, but "anything more would have made me feel like I was selling a baby." She added, "If you think about it, I could have made more at work." Another woman said she was not paid enough for all that she suffered. On the other hand, she shrank from the idea of putting a price on a baby. There isn't a fair price for a baby," she insisted. Still, she said $20,000 would have been preferable to $10,000.

Yet a third woman added, "I feel that the service I rendered should have been paid for. I think the price could have been higher and I also think that no matter how high the price went, people would still pay to have a child of their own."

When all was said and done, and the baby was in the hands of the adoptive couple, surrogate mothers reportedly experienced a variety of emotions. At the positive end of the scale, many of the women surveyed for this book said they walked away with a glow born of having performed a special act. At the negative end, these women experienced everything from letdown after an exciting experience to regret at having to give away the baby of their dreams. But even a surrogate mother who claimed to have had a miserable experience found that making others happy was "the one positive aspect of surrogate parenting."

Then there were the women for whom surrogacy was so special that none of the negative things that happened to them seemed to matter. One surrogate was temporarily transferred from her job as an X-ray technician and placed in another department because her boss feared liability if the baby was born with a birth defect. To make matters worse, her parents were highly critical of her surrogacy. But none of these problems discouraged her. "Nobody can imagine the feeling you have to be able to give someone a child that they may never have gotten if it wasn't for me," she said. When she received her payment she took her family to Disney World with the money. "The happiness of my children was also something that made it all worthwhile. We would never have been able to do that if it wasn't for what I did," she affirmed.

And although many find it hard to believe, the majority of

surrogates interviewed were willing to do it again. More than half of the California women said they would act as surrogates a second or even a third time, but only for the same couple. Among the reasons the women gave for refusing a repeat surrogacy were age and the fear that the impact of another surrogate pregnancy might have some deleterious effect on their marriages and families. And there were surrogates who either had mixed emotions about their surrogacy experience or simply had no interest in a repeat performance. Some of the women regarded being a surrogate mother as the most important contribution of their lives. To serve as a surrogate more than once would cheapen their gift they reasoned. "I have done the most important thing I will ever do, but I won't do it again," said one surrogate.

For most of the women who chose to serve as surrogates more than once, the experience was close to being perfect each time. There was nothing they would have changed the second or third time around. Others said they would be willing to bear a child for strangers again only if they could change the contract, meet the couple, or be part of a surrogate support group. And once again, California surrogates had their own wish list. Only a solid relationship with the couple in question would induce the majority of these women to act as surrogates a second time. Several surrogates also said they would not consider repeat surrogacies unless they received some assurance that the physical aspects of the procedure—insemination, conception, and pregnancy—would go more smoothly.

If any single individual can be said to understand the psyche of women who become surrogate mothers, it's Hilary Hanafin, the staff psychologist at the Center of Surrogate Parenting in Los Angeles. Hanafin, who wrote her doctoral dissertation on surrogacy, set up the surrogate-mother counseling group at the center and handles all the center's screening of surrogates and couples. In the course of the screening process she rejects 90 percent of the women who apply to be surrogate mothers. Those she accepts are similar to the women who were surveyed for this book—mothers who tend to "find great pleasure in being pregnant and get a lot of pleasure out of helping other people." Hanafin added, "Whether they're acting out of psychological need or personal satisfaction, it's not surprising to find women in the helping professions. Women who tend to have more potential than they've been able to manifest because of psychological issues, family, or societal reasons. Often women who wanted to do something further, but something got in the way. Surrogate parenting allows them to feel special."

Hanafin admits that these same tendencies can be pathological if carried to the extreme—that there can be something wrong with a woman who denies her own needs and gives solely to others. On two occasions she has rejected women who described themselves as the sort of people to whom others always came with their problems. She can tell from their case histories that these women are in the habit of suppressing their needs to those of others. "We turn down women with a martyr syndrome—whose sense of self is lost," she said. This is not to say that Hanafin frowns upon altruistic tendencies. On the contrary, she considers it "healthy when a surrogate can show she enjoys doing for others but can still put herself first if need be." She went on to say that for these women "there is still satisfaction in giving to others, but it is not based on low self-esteem. The psychological testing we do helps indicate that. The women in the group [surrogate-mother counseling group] are generally other-centered."

In order for surrogacy to be a rewarding, self-satisfying experience for them, Hanafin feels the women involved need support from those closest to them. She will not accept women as surrogates unless that "significant other gives 100 percent support to the process." Spouses and boyfriends of prospective surrogates must submit to an interview, meet the couple, and attend a support group session.

Only when their support is determined to be genuine will the women involved be accepted into her program. Hanafin also looks for women who can stand up to the constant stream of comments and criticism from outsiders (surrogate mothers) often face. "All surrogates must struggle with the fact that other people just don't understand. They're constantly being judged. This is true of anyone who does anything controversial," she affirmed.

According to Hanafin the first thing a surrogate has to deal with—even earlier than the couple—is how family, friends, and coworkers will respond. "This is much more critical, more imminent, for a surrogate," she said. Then there's the question of what to tell older children and when? Will it jeopardize jobs, relationships?" Hanafin has found that negative comments or implied negative comments from outsiders are common. "Women who get a lot of negative feedback up front typically won't go forward with it," she said. "We've had surrogates who've had problems with husbands, boyfriends, and jobs which has made it difficult. We've had women with unaccepting mothers and fathers who just wouldn't talk about it." If the staff at the Los Angeles center feels that criticism from outsiders and family is unwarranted, they sometimes advise the women involved in their program to ignore it. Hanafin cited the case of a woman whose mother violently objected to her becoming a surrogate. Knowing the younger woman's history, she said, the staff "felt this wasn't a bad thing for her." She added, "We felt it was a real step for her; something uncomfortable and painful, but a growth process."

Hanafin is also wary of women who may be too judgmental or too curious about the adoptive couple. "If they only want a couple of a certain age, religion, or money bracket, they shouldn't be in a surrogate program," she said. "They can be specific, but not so specific that the couple won't meet their expectations." Because roughly two-thirds of the surrogates in her program have been raised as Christians—

Hanafin reported that only a handful of black, Asian or Jewish women apply—and couples tend to come from more varied religious backgrounds, Hanafin feels it is important that surrogates be able to accept the possibility that a child be reared in another faith or culture. If they cannot or have trouble accepting this fact they may be rejected.

Once they have been admitted into the Los Angeles surrogate parenting program, women who serve as surrogate mothers become immersed in a different world—one with its own list of stresses and strains. Hanafin and her colleagues have done pioneering work in identifying the kinds of issues surrogates may face and in confronting them head-on before they become major problems. She says one of the purposes of the surrogate support group is to help these women "determine who is saying what." Negative comments may be coming from a jealous girl friend, and this, she says "is different from a girl friend who finds the idea of surrogacy unsettling because she has had an abortion. We tell the surrogates to explore where people are coming from. If they want to continue, we try to play a supportive role."

What to tell their own children is another issue of major concern for many surrogates in Hanafin's program. She encourages the women to open and honest about their actions, to tell their children about the couple. A meeting between the couple and the surrogate's children is considered ideal. In the absence of a meeting, however, Hanafin suggests that surrogates be "consistent and patient" in explaining their actions to her children." To protect their children from outside comment, she recommends that her surrogates contact their children's teachers and explain the program "so they won't say inappropriate things." She also suggests that they do the same regarding the other adults in the children's lives.

Hanafin has found that a surrogate also needs assistance in conceptualizing the child she is carrying for others and in determining how to categorize her pregnancy. They must determine whether the child is theirs, a shared child prenatally, or the couple's child. "Most surrogates think of it as the couple's child because they only conceived the child through a commitment and relationship with the couple," she said. "This happens without any coaching from the center. We don't encourage this attitude, confront it, or challenge it if that's the way they've chosen to cope with it. If they see the child as shared, that's okay. If they think of it as their's, then we would look at the situation closely. No doubt it would be harder for a surrogate mother to relinquish the child under those circumstances."

Like couples, surrogates, too, can have a difficult time with the waiting that is such an unavoidable part of the surrogacy process. During the course of their pregnancy many surrogates begin worrying that their bodies will fail them, thus becoming more attuned to the feelings of the infertile couples who have turned to them for assistance. Hanafin cautions her surrogates against putting "inordinate amounts of pressure on themselves and their bodies to perform." For the surrogates' sake, she asks couples to maintain some sort of contact during the pregnancy. Most surrogates, she said, "just want to get together during that time. They feel they could let go better if the couple would be a part of their lives for nine months. If the couple doesn't express joy during the pregnancy, it's harder on the surrogate."

According to Hanafin, what surrogates find most disturbing—"what they don't even want to hear"—is that the couple still questions their motives after all they've done. "Here's this woman wanting to do something so special, setting aside her own life, and the couple still doesn't believe or trust her completely," she explained. She tries to shield the surrogate mothers in her program from their couples' anxiety. At the same time, she is sympathetic to the couples and the tensions they must undergo during the surrogacy process. An advocate of legalizing surrogate parenting, Hanafin believes that binding contracts will go a long way toward clearing up the concerns exhibited by many of the couples with whom she has worked. "It would be nice if we didn't have to prove this is okay," she said.

Then there is the issue of the separation process. Hanafin has found that just as the relationship between surrogates and couples comes to an end, it often becomes most intense. At this point she feels it is appropriate for the surrogate to conceptualize the child as the couple's and begin to anticipate with relief the end of her pregnancy and the return to a normal life for herself and her family. "Like any pregnant lady, she's taken on a major project that's as practical as it is emotional." According to Hanafin much of the sadness experienced at this stage usually revolves around the surrogate having to say good-bye to being a surrogate—saying good-bye to all the excitement and attention that are a potential part of the role. She has found that surrogates often have a harder time saying good-bye to the couple than to the baby because their feelings of attachment are usually focused on the couple. Of course, giving up the child can be difficult. But Hanafin has found that most surrogates feel toward the child as they would toward a niece or nephew. "And I hear this without prompting them," she said. "They just don't feel that this baby belongs in their home. We've even had several surrogates express surprise that the baby looked like them. That's how much they've denied their contribution to the process. And as much concern as they have for the newborn, most just want to go home to their own children."

Still, for many surrogate mothers the hospital experience and the short time with the baby have proved to be the highlight of their experience. Especially delightful for most, according to Hanafin, was actually getting to see the couple with the baby they had helped to produce. "We hear this over and over. We also hear feelings of being very proud and very impressed with themselves." Although many surrogate mothers worry about not producing a healthy, "perfect" baby, as of this writing there have been no babies born with birth defects or other problems in Hanafin's Los Angeles program. Quite frankly, Hanafin feels lucky she has not had to deal with "the guilt over unhealthy babies" and knows this is an issue everyone at the center will have to face someday.

Despite the prevailing attitude of good-natured acceptance, however, Hanafin has noted that relinquishment time isn't always a joyous occasion. This is especially true if a woman's motive for becoming a surrogate has to do with mitigating the guilt of a past adoption or abortion. Memories of such an event can surface at the time of relinquishment, which Hanafin said "may make them remember the baby they gave up for adoption or aborted."

During the course of postpartum counseling, Hanafin has discovered that women who come to surrogate parenting in search of a special experience usually have a harder time walking away than do those who come into it for other reasons. "Sometimes they hang on to the program and decide to do it again. Others do a reevaluation and decide to make this their last pregnancy. There is the potential for sadness if the sex of the child relinquished was the one a woman wanted for her family," Hanafin said. And dealing with the external world could be just as difficult postpartum as it was at earlier stages of the surrogacy, she found. Former surrogate mothers have told Hanafin that people approached them on a regular basis and asked them how they were really feeling. What bothered the women, according to Hanafin, was the implication "that they were having more pain and grief than they revealed. This hurt," she explained, "because it showed them that their friends and families weren't accepting the beauty of what they were doing. They felt that people were watching and waiting for them to break down and they get really tired of it."

Hanafin said she counsels her surrogates to realize that their actions have been personal, may be difficult to explain to others, and that they themselves are fine no matter what others think. Some surrogates have coped with the world's lack of understanding by holding onto the relationship they developed with their couples. Others have continued to attend the center's group sessions for the social contact and support they offer. However, Hanafin has found that most surrogates maintain only minimal contact with their couples following the birth. Although she hasn't conducted a study on this aspect of surrogate parenting, she said there have been only four or five surrogates and couples—"a very low percentage"—who chose to maintain close contact after the birth.

Despite the enormous potential for emotional upset inherent in surrogacy, Hanafin said she has yet to meet a woman who regretted acting as a surrogate mother. Two former surrogates have told her that the process was harder than they thought it would be, and two others wondered whether they had done the right thing. But these regrets were usually fleeting. "I don't know of any cases of long-term regrets or depression, she said. "I have had surrogates who wished things had ended differently; who would have liked more contact with the baby, or some pictures." More often, though, Hanafin has encountered former surrogates who felt guilty at having had less attachment to the child than they had expected. "They wanted to know if this was all right; whether they were all right," she said.

In answer to one of society's most pointed criticisms, Hanafin does not believe that centers like hers are fostering a "breeder class" of women. For most women, she said, surrogacy is a one-time thing: "We're not vending machines popping out kids in mass quantities. They're doing something special once in their life. We don't even describe this as a role."

At the Center for Reproductive Alternatives in Northern California, Lyn Brown has found that most of the surrogate mothers she has encountered are altruistic in the sense that they "want to contribute something to make the world a better place." Generally "nurturing, supermom types" with children of their own, she says "they understand a lot of the principles that are important for child development. These women believe in the future; that the world has a future and it's the kids." Brown urges anyone involved in surrogate parenting to seek legal guidance and psychological counseling. "What they're doing is very unique and it helps for everyone, especially the surrogates, to be part of a support group," she said. The surrogates she has encountered "are very clear about their role." What they're not so clear about is the time-consuming nature of the process and the need for patience. "The main thing we have to counsel them about is not expecting to conceive the first time; that it can take six months. That's one of the things that drives them crazy she said. "The period from the first legal meeting until the start of insemination and from the start of insemination to conception can be stressful for everyone."

Brown, too, recommends openness about the process between the surrogate and her family and the surrogate and the couple. "Secrecy is poisonous," she affirmed. She also suggests that the surrogate and the couple work together as a team. Most of the surrogates in her program have expressed a preference for the involvement of the adoptive mother in the pregnancy, even to the extent of attending Lamaze classes and being in the delivery room. If a prospective mother doesn't want contact with the couple, she is advised to try another program. Brown feels that anonymity creates too many problems. As far as she's concerned, getting strangers together "doesn't create problems, it creates a support network." As for the actual relinquishing of the child, Brown advises surrogates to work out whatever scenario they prefer with their couple. Additional support is provided in the surrogate counseling group. "Before or after delivery, if there's a problem with being ambivalent, they have access to the staff psychologist," she said.

For the most part, Brown said she has seen little ambivalence among the women in their program. "You never hear a surrogate saying 'my child.' They fully believe they're carrying the child for someone else. You usually hear this before insemination." Brown has pointed out that most surrogates don't want another child to raise. "I think these women are very exceptional. I love their outlook on life. They're positive people. I admire them," she concluded.

And Jan Sutton, who has come in contact with about as many surrogate mothers as anyone in the field, considers her peers to be very loving, caring people: "They may come from different walks of life and have different life-styles, but they believe in giving others the happiness of a child—something they couldn't experience otherwise. They're just the neatest people. I haven't met one I didn't like."

# 3

## THE INTERMEDIARIES

# 7 | A Clinic Director's Perspective

If directors of surrogate parenting clinics are a rare breed, then Elaine Silver is a maverick among mavericks. In general, the field is dominated by lawyers, doctors, and psychologists who approach surrogate parenting from a businesslike point of view. Some are more caring than others, some are more sensitive. But as a whole their objective is to match couples with surrogates, create babies, pay the bills, recoup some profit, and, if all goes well, incur no liability.

As a woman who battled infertility and eventually had a child via surrogacy, Elaine Silver has firsthand knowledge of the process. She knows the depth of longing that drives infertile couples to try almost any alternative that will bring them a child. And she knows the tremendous rewards surrogacy has to offer. In addition to being a psychiatric social worker by training, Elaine believes her own experience with surrogacy has given her a unique empathy for all parties involved in surrogate parenting. For better or worse, she has been governed more by that empathy than by any real inter-

est in the surrogate parenting program as a business—
sometimes to the detriment of her pocketbook. To her, the
matching of a surrogate with an infertile couple is akin to a
religious act. She once said she would prefer that no money
changed hands during the process because the exchange
"lessens the surrogate's gift."

To understand Elaine is to place her in the context of the
sixties, when thousands of young people flocked into the
social service fields with a dream of making the world a better place. Elaine, who is now in her mid-thirties, was one of
those thousands. Bringing babies to infertile couples has
been her way of improving society. It has also been a means
of resolving her own infertility. For Elaine is one of those
women who from their teenage years have a gut feeling that
they won't be able to have children. The first, real signs of
her infertility cropped up in 1973 when she suffered a miscarriage. After visiting several specialists, Elaine was told
that she had chronic endometriosis, a scarring of the uterine
wall that makes it difficult for a fertilized egg to take hold
and develop.

As a young woman in her early twenties, Elaine was not
prepared to accept a life sentence of infertility and have her
dream of a large family shattered. She had no way of knowing that her fertility problems would eventually lead her to a
career on the fringes of reproductive science. "I was twenty-
three years old. I'd heard all these horror stories from wom-
en who at thirty-one and thirty-two were trying to get pregnant for the first time. But at twenty-three you never expect
that kind of problem," she said, looking back. Devastated
by the miscarriage—but unable to give up her dream of having children—Elaine immediately put her name on an
adoption list to "compensate for the loss." This move alien-
ated her husband, who had been an adopted child. Reluc-
tant to relive that experience by adopting children of his
own, he pushed Elaine to continue trying to have a baby
naturally. She went along for six years.

"If emotionally, on some level, I gave up hope, I never gave up medically. When there's hope it's horrible to give up, Elaine said, remembering how easily she got pregnant. It seemed crazy to stop trying when she knew she was producing eggs that could be fertilized. But the next pregnancy ended in miscarriage, as did the four that followed. With each succeeding pregnancy the uterine scarring worsened. Doctors told Elaine a lot of things, including the fact that she hadn't given herself time to heal. Five specialists later she agreed to try experimental drugs. Nothing helped.

In 1976, halfway through her battle with infertility, Elaine and her husband were able to adopt a baby boy. Her husband had relented and Elaine, who had just miscarried a baby boy, felt this adoption was fated. What proved equally eventful was the job she took not long after bringing Michael home—a job working on a hot line for pregnant teenagers. Through the hot line Elaine began to do a lot of adoption-related counseling. After a few months a social worker told her she was perfectly suited for the work.

In 1977 the woman arranged through the agency to send Elaine to Yeshiva University in New York to earn her master's in social work. The arrangement was ideal academically but rough on Elaine's homelife. For two years and three summers she lived in New York from June through August and then did practical social work with the agency at home during the rest of the year. Although she commuted on weekends during the summer, this wasn't satisfactory for her husband. He was left at home to care for a child toward whom he was at best ambivalent. With each miscarriage he had become increasingly morose. Unlike Elaine, he could not accept an alternative to their infertility. The introduction of an adopted child into their lives only made him "more depressed and withdrawn." While she saw graduate school as a means to a career she enjoyed, he felt betrayed.

As Elaine's career advanced she found her homelife more and more of a shambles. In the summer of 1978 she and her husband agreed to a trial separation. What brought the two back together that September was notification that they were at the top of the list at local adoption agency. "Being someone who didn't give up I said 'let's try'," she recalled. "We'd been in therapy for five years. I didn't want to believe this was the end of the relationship." Ruth was adopted in January 1979 as a newborn just as Michael was going through the terrible twos. Not long after the adoption, Elaine accepted a job placement at a mental health center. Although this position involved longer hours than her previous job had, she felt she would develop new therapeutic skills. As if this wasn't enough, she was writing her master's thesis. With Elaine becoming increasingly involved in her career, her husband fell apart. She had no choice but to persevere. She received her master's degree that summer, accepted a full-time job at the mental health center in the fall of 1979, and, now able to support herself, asked her husband for a divorce. Both finally agreed that they were incompatible.

Her infertility might have precipitated the crisis in Elaine's marriage, but she came to see this as only part of a larger problem. "Here I was with two small children, I had a job, I'd just bought a house, and when people asked why I was getting a divorce I said if I was going to be the one giving 100 percent, I'd rather be alone. I was alone anyway."

There's nothing easy about divorce, especially when you're a divorced mother of two small children. But at least Elaine didn't have to live with the stress of an unhappy relationship. And with divorce came a new relationship and a new career. Her friendship with her supervisor—"a warm, supportive man named John"—eventually evolved into a romance. But from the start, children were an issue. Although John cared for Elaine's adopted children, he hoped they could have children of their own. Elaine's fears were resurrected when she became pregnant by John and miscarried. This was one pregnancy and one miscarriage too many. Deciding to have a hysterectomy, Elaine told her fiancé that she "couldn't live her life as a sick person who isn't really a sick person when I could be healthy. I had to physically and emotionally call it quits," she said. When they were married in October 1982, Elaine and John toyed with the idea of adopting a child together. But when Elaine learned of a surrogate parenting center operating on the East Coast, she became enthralled with the idea of turning to another woman to bear their child. On a whim, she called up the director. That call changed the course of her life in more ways than one.

After learning about Elaine's training—especially her adoption experience—the director of the clinic, Barbara, invited her for a visit. She was interested in the idea of setting up a franchise in New England and thought Elaine might be the perfect person to run it. Intrigued by the possibilities unfolding before her, Elaine took the trip. And what an amazing trip it was. In Barbara's office she was able to witness, firsthand, the matching of infertile couples with women who had agreed to bear their children. She was overwhelmed by this new world, by these new opportunities, and very much wanted to be a part of this process—part of a revolution in reproductive techniques.

Both women saw in each other characteristics and skills the other lacked. Barbara had business know-how, "a known name, and clout." Elaine was a social worker with a good deal of therapeutic experience. It felt like such a good match that at the end of her visit Barbara asked Elaine to open a New England branch of her surrogate parenting clinic. Barbara agreed to teach Elaine all she knew about screening surrogates and couples as well as other procedural elements of surrogate parenting. Privately, Elaine hoped she could inject a little personal touch into the operation. The New England franchise opened in August 1983. But almost from the start, Elaine chafed at the rules that had been set up by the home office. She had trouble with the business-first attitude of the other office, and with the insistence on maintaining strict anonymity between surrogates and couples.

It soon became apparent to Elaine that she and Barbara had very different personal styles. Elaine wanted "adults to make up their own minds about how to operate." She wanted surrogate parenting to be more than a business deal. Over the next two years these stylistic differences deepened into a major schism. By the spring of 1985 Barbara asked for Elaine's resignation. (At her office several years after the split, Barbara said she felt she and Elaine were incompatible as business partners. A staunch businesswoman, she said she thought Elaine took too many risks. She was afraid Elaine's attitude would lead to some major catastrophe—the "Baby M" case, for example.)

In the settlement worked out between the lawyers for both women, Elaine agreed not to compete with Barbara for six months. She took on no new clients from June 1985 until December. It was a time of soul-searching. For a while Elaine wasn't even certain she would stay in the business. She needed time to think things over and recoup financially from the more than $7,000 bank loan she had taken out to cover fee disputes. There was one positive outcome of this period—the birth by surrogate mother of Elaine's son David.

Prior to the business split-up, the home office had found a surrogate mother for Elaine and John, and artificial insemination had been arranged. Because of the distance and expense, John flew out for the insemination alone. Although Elaine now encourages both couples to participate in the insemination process, at the time she had no regrets about staying at home. Like Linda McRobbie, she felt relieved to have someone else handle the pressure. And as far as Elaine was concerned, her son was conceived because she and her husband wanted a child. "He was 100 percent ours in that way. I never felt left out of that. Sure, I would have liked to have been a part of the ejaculations, but it was too expensive," she said later.

As soon as her husband went through with the first insemination attempt, Elaine found herself in the incongruous position of being surrogate parenting director to clients while she, too, was part of a couple participating in a surrogate parenting program. It was incongruous but, invaluable in helping her to understand the emotions involved in the process. For example, she now knew from personal experience how excruciating it was to wait for news about your surrogate and the conception. When their surrogate mother, Carol, did conceive seven months later, Elaine suffered the familiar pangs of sadness at her inability to bear a child and found it as difficult as her clients to be an "expectant" mother while having had virtually no involvement in the pregnancy. As a clinic director and psychiatric social worker, Elaine was able to work with her emotions. She compensated for her own lack of involvement by "never forgetting that this woman was bearing us a child."

Elaine and John's experience with surrogacy was complicated by the split-up of the two surrogate parenting centers. Barbara had stipulated that they be treated like any other couple and insisted that the home office handle their case. Due to the anonymity rule and tension between the offices, Elaine had less contact with Carol than she would have liked. When the actual breakup took place in June, Elaine's attorney called Carol and inquired whether she would like to work directly with Elaine and John. The woman—who was physically fine but disturbed by all the confusion—agreed to a meeting and to hand control of her case over to Elaine. Elaine found it wonderful to meet Carol and her husband that July. Carol was then five months pregnant. They discussed the birth and pending delivery in November. Elaine couldn't get over being "allowed to experience the pregnancy." And she remained in almost constant communication, learning from Carol when the fetus moved for the first time and that an ultrasound had revealed she was carrying a boy, whom Elaine and John called David.

From that point on, Carol's pregnancy proved a blueprint for all others that Elaine would later administer. (The McRobbies were affected by this change in policy on anonymity midstream.) She dropped all notions of anonymity and worked hard to build a trusting, though distant, relationship with her surrogate mother. As Carol lived in another state, Elaine found it helpful to compare notes with a close friend who was pregnant and due around the same time. "Basically, I was very proud of what was going on, very excited. That Halloween my husband and I went to a Halloween party as a pregnant couple. Only we were both pregnant, which I felt was equal."

Like other couples, Elaine and John learned to be careful of what they said about the surrogate birth, limiting conversations on the subject to an occasional store clerk, close friends, and family. Although the feedback was generally positive, they were aware that many people in the world did not view surrogate parenting as they did. "Anytime you meet new people and tell them about surrogate parenting, you open a can of worms," Elaine discovered, a message she passed on to others involved in her program. "You have to be careful about anonymity. You don't want the child pointed out later as a surrogate baby," she cautioned.

One of the things that had disturbed Elaine about the home office procedures was the rule banning couples from the labor room. As Carol's due date neared, she made arrangements for herself and John to be present at the delivery. Carol's ready agreement made Elaine feel more secure than ever that her surrogate mother would have no problems relinquishing the baby. Several weeks before the due date of November 11, Elaine, John, and the older children took a family trip to Disneyworld. "It was our last trip as a foursome, Elaine said, looking back. "We all talked of David and what would be happening." It was while they were in Florida that Elaine learned that the fetus was breech. There was some question of the need to perform a cesarean section. Elaine became anxious and began to lobby for a C-section and Carol went along, but the doctor said no. He wanted to give it another few days.

The "few days" became two weeks. This doctor subscribed to the notion that babies come when they're ready. Nothing happened until the night before Thanksgiving. Just as Elaine popped some baked goods into the oven, the call came in that Carol was in labor. She and John left the two children with relatives and sped to the hospital. David was born at 2:34 A.M. Exactly three minutes later, Elaine and John were able to hold their baby boy for the first time. Elaine recalled standing there holding the baby and "just crying, and crying and crying."

The relinquishment proceedings took place the next day, along with a visit to Carol. Although Elaine had no problems with her surrogate mother spending time with the baby, Carol chose not to do so. "She felt she had said goodbye to him. She knew she would have contact with him through us," Elaine explained. "She had distanced herself with the idea that this was our baby. Besides, she felt a closeness to our family."

Elaine spoke to Carol every day during the first month after the birth, in part out of personal concern and in part as clinic director. She saw Carol once that summer after David was born and the first year talked to her about him monthly. She assumes she "will always have some contact around the holidays and on birthdays." Several weeks after the birth Carol wrote thanking her and John for making it possible for her to be a surrogate mother. "She felt that if she had died right then, she would have done something special. I couldn't believe this woman was thanking us for this gift of life. When I think of Carol it really angers me when couples won't spend money [on their surrogates]. I go through the ceiling, especially when they say $10,000 for the surrogate is enough, to compensate them for all their efforts."

When David was six months old, Elaine and her husband

went through the legalities of formal adoption. She found this to be one of the most difficult aspects of the surrogate parenting process. "Nervous as hell that the judge would deny the adoption and sweating bullets," she and her family prepared for their court appearance. As it turned out, they were in the judge's chambers for about thirty seconds. The documents, previously signed, sat before him. Would he petition for another six months' trial period or sign David over to them for life? With little fanfare, the judge said David was theirs.

Thinking back on the pregnancy, birth, and adoption Elaine has credited her ongoing work with other surrogates and couples with helping her to survive the turmoil of those months. From their experiences she was able to reap the benefits of having been through it before. Although she does not feel that all clinic directors must live the process themselves in order to guide others, Elaine does feel that David's birth made her particularly well equipped to anticipate the needs of others and that she has a deeper insight than most into the problems that many couples will encounter during the course of their surrogate parenting experience. If there is any aspect of surrogate parenting that Elaine found disturbing as she experienced it, it is anonymity between couples and surrogates. For her, anonymity produces a pervasive sense of vulnerability that is unnecessary. Until Carol actually agreed to reveal herself and work with Elaine, Elaine feared she would be upset by all the changes between clinics and not want to work openly together on the pregnancy and birth. "It was supposed to be anonymous. I didn't know how she would feel about breaking that rule," she said.

One of the most positive aspects of David's birth by surrogacy has been its role in helping Elaine to resolve her own infertility. She feels that the other wonderful aspect of surrogacy is that it allows people to have children when they're emotionally ready to do so. "One of the horrible aspects of infertility," she said, "is the fact that people have to keep trying and trying to have kids whether they're ready or not. They're always planning to have a baby; it becomes a constant state of wanting a baby. With adoption I found I wasn't always ready when the agency was, but you're not about to turn down a child."

David's birth came toward the end of Elaine's six months in professional limbo, during which she had plenty of time to reflect on how she would operate her own clinic. When December 1985 came around and she decided to resume operation of the clinic under her own direction, she realized that her personal surrogate parenting experience had radically changed her professional approach to the process. As was previously mentioned the McRobbies were greatly affected by these policy changes, the first and most important which was to allow contact between the surrogates and their couples. As adults, Elaine felt they should have the option of deciding whether to meet one another. She made sure everyone already enrolled in the program understood the positive and negative aspects of direct communication; and eight couples and surrogates then under contract opted for contact. According to Elaine, those couples felt contact would give them more control over the process. Some of them told Elaine that they would feel more relaxed if they knew from their surrogate mother what she was doing, and they thought she would have an easier time relinquishing if she knew them. They felt they would be able to share in the pregnancy, see the ultrasounds, be in the delivery room.

Although she personally favors contact, Elaine also understands what some people regard as the negative aspects of this approach. Knowing one another can make it more difficult for both surrogates and couples to "break the ties." And, according to Elaine, many infertile couples don't want an ongoing relationship with the surrogate. They want to take the baby and get on with their lives—a fact that most surrogates understand and handle well. Elaine has found

that when surrogates get to know their couples they sometimes complain to them about their condition or emotions
rather than going to her. Not all couples want to hear about
nausea and discomfort, it seems. "Although they want to be
involved, if there's any complaining they want it to go to
me," she explained.

It's Elaine's experience that most surrogates simply want
to feel appreciated. Most also favor some contact with their
couple, because at the very least they can gain reassurance
that the baby is going to a loving set of parents. Although
Elaine won't insist on a relationship between a couple and
their surrogate mother, after David's birth she did urge couples to give their surrogates more consideration and respect.
Elaine also determined to provide surrogates they could respect. Tightening her screening process, she no longer allowed unmarried women into the program, welfare mothers, or someone with even a hint of a criminal past. "I tend
now to be harder on couples than I ought or need to be because of how eternally grateful I feel toward our surrogate. I
especially want the adoptive mother to see her surrogate as
an ally, not an enemy. This is a woman who did something
wonderful for them [the couple]. That's how I viewed Carol.
I think she's about the most wonderful person who walks
the face of the earth," she said.

Once the baby is born Elaine has found that many couples—especially those who have not resolved their infertility—want to distance themselves from both the surrogate
and the clinic. "At that juncture," said Elaine, "they want to
pretend that there was no one else involved in the birth of
their baby. Often the fear is there, too, that the surrogate
will want to take back the baby. I understand the fear, and it
is a valid one. The couples wonder at what point the connection with the surrogate really ends. My feeling is that
there has to be an agreement between both sides made long
before the baby is born that stipulates when this will be. I
know that in a lot of my cases this wasn't so, and I've

changed the agreement to make it more solid; to make sure all parties are certain what will happen in the end. This has been an issue."

Elaine has noted that surrogates are equally hurt by the couples' fear of losing the baby—a fear she believes could be easily remedied by legalization of the process and recognition of the adoptive parents as the legal parents from conception. "I feel badly for many surrogates who are later deserted by couples. I often feel the couples don't respect them. The surrogates can't understand the fear on the couples' part. Seeing a picture of the child, for instance, wouldn't make any of them want to take the child back."

In general, most couples agree to send pictures to surrogates within a year after the birth, which Elaine feels is a "reasonable time for closure." She added, "The baby is a different baby by the end of the year. It seems to be everyone's feeling that this would be the final good-bye." As for her own continued contact with surrogates and couples, Elaine goes case by case. She's in daily contact with the surrogate for the first month after delivery. She usually leaves the couple alone for the first week to give them some time "to glow." She then calls the couple at least once afterward. At the end of six months she and the couple usually have some contact to make preparations for the adoption. But for the most part, Elaine hears more from her surrogates than from her couples because the couples usually want to get on with their lives. Everyone who has ever participated in Elaine's program (there were seventeen births by the fall of 1986) receives a card at Christmas.

Along with the changes in procedure, after December 1985 Elaine altered her business practices as well. First she changed her fee system. Instead of accepting a $10,000 fee from a couple up front and then locating a surrogate—sometimes a lengthy process—she decided to charge the couple only when she had an available surrogate and a signed contract by both parties. As for the contract, she felt it was too open-ended. In 1986 she determined that each couple and their surrogate should negotiate up front "each dime" of the expenses above and beyond the clinic and surrogate fees. Everything incurred in travel, medical expenses, postpartum health care, or day care for the surrogate's children—whatever each threesome decided—had to be put in writing.

For many reasons the financial aspect of surrogate parenting has always bothered Elaine. "I hate to put a financial figure on what the surrogate is doing," she said. "Somehow that lessens the gift. I feel the same about my fee. But let's be realistic, nothing is gratis. Nor should this be." Elaine's clients expect her to be available twenty-four hours a day, seven days a week: "They expect the moon. I try to be available, and it's taken a large toll. I have a hard time setting limits because I have an aversion to the business part. But I couldn't do this if I made it more like a business. My husband urges me all the time to be more businesslike, to protect myself more. People expect it. Yet I don't see surrogate parenting as a business deal, and I don't see this as a job."

Having been in business for about three years as of the fall of 1986, Elaine said she saw her clinic and her personal situation evolving. As time went on, she said she could see her own role changing as she became more of a consultant. She could see herself aiding surrogates and couples who have already found each other and have come to her for psychological counseling or to gain "an understanding of the issues." She has talked with people who have arranged a surrogate agreement on their own and always advises them to contact a specialist in this: "People are naive. They assume nothing will go wrong. Things do go wrong and will go wrong. It's nice for things to be discussed ahead of time so no one is shocked." Would she ever choose to leave the surrogate parenting business? "I've had lots of pressure to give it up," Elaine answered. "But as long as there is an available surrogate, I'm in it."

# 8 | Surrogate Parenting Clinics: A National Survey

Judging from the activities of surrogate parenting clinics and centers nationwide, surrogate parenting is beginning to come into its own. In some parts of the country—California, Kansas, and Kentucky, for example—the procedure is well established if not yet part of the mainstream health-care network. Although the Michigan lawyer Noel Keane opened up the first surrogate parenting operation in the mid-1970s, surrogate parenting clinics and centers did not begin to proliferate until 1980.

As stated in Chapter Four, an estimated 12,000 to 15,000 infertile couples contacted these centers between 1980 and 1987 to express their interest in surrogate parenting. And although exact statistics are impossible to gather because many clinics either do not keep figures or refuse to release them, by early 1987 as many as 600 babies had been born to infertile couples making use of these centers. As public awareness of the procedure increases, fertility experts expect this number to grow. The controversial "Baby M" case, which came to national attention in 1986, did much to awaken Americans to the issues surrounding surrogate parenting. In January 1987 *Newsweek* magazine published a poll indicating that 61 percent of its sample knew about surrogate parenting and were aware of this case. Just as important, a majority of those surveyed supported the process as a viable alternative for infertile women or women who might suffer medically from bearing children.

Because clinics try to attract a large number of surrogates to meet the needs of the couples on their roster, the survey conducted for this book indicates that about four times as many potential surrogate mothers had contact with clinics as couples between 1980 and 1987. In 1986—the year data for this book was collected—clinic directors talked with about 4,300 women who were interested in becoming surrogate mothers and accepted a little less than half of these for participation in their programs. They estimated that at least 20,000 to 25,000 women nationwide contacted their programs from 1980 to 1987 to inquire about becoming surrogate mothers.

A surprising number of surrogate parenting clinics have come and gone since 1980. In her 1984 book *New Conceptions*, Lori B. Andrews published a list of twenty-four surrogate parenting clinics located in a variety of states across the country. Three years later just under half of the clinics she listed were no longer in existence, though several new clinics had been established through the creation of franchises or the breakup of partnerships. (The two former clinic directors who could be reached—the others had closed up shop, giving no return address or phone number—said they weren't able to make it financially.) At the time of this writing California had the largest number of clinics, with centers in Beverly Hills, San Clemente, San Francisco, Pleasant Hills, and at least two in Los Angeles. Nationwide, other clinics were found in Louisville, Kentucky; Topeka, Kansas; Chevy Chase, Maryland; Springfield, Massachusetts; Dearborn, Michigan; New York City; and Portland, Oregon. The clinics that had gone out of business by the mid-1980s were located in Costa Mesa, California; Denver, Colorado; Columbia, Maryland; Livonia, Michigan; East Greenbush, Jamaica, and Medford, New York; Columbus, Ohio; Philadelphia, Pennsylvania; and Kirkland, Washington.

As of early 1987, the South had virtually no widely recognized surrogate parenting clinics outside of Kentucky. Surrogate parenting, however, was being practiced in Florida through the assistance of attorneys. The Midwest was only lightly represented, and fewer clinics existed on the East Coast than on the West Coast. California clinic owners and directors reported that a solid proportion of their business came from clients in the Southwest, especially Texas. They also reported handling clients from the Orient and Europe.

If few surrogate parenting clinics or centers existed in the nation's southern tier at that time, it was not for lack of interest. Individuals from Georgia, Oklahoma, and Kentucky responded to a nationwide appeal for research subjects released for this project by the Newspaper Enterprise Association. Some were merely curious about the surrogate parenting process, but others sought information with the intent of opening their own clinics or becoming surrogates. On a nationwide basis clinics that managed to survive the infancy of the phenomenon were well established and thriving in 1987. Some, including the Hagar Institute in Topeka, Kansas, had established clinics in other states. Others, such as the Center of Surrogate Parenting in Beverly Hills, California, had expanded their staff to the point of maintaining a full-time psychologist and hiring a public relations firm.

What many of the successful clinics were found to have in common was a founder who had previously worked in the fields of law, medicine, psychology, social work, or education. Many of them chose to maintain their basic practices and hire others to operate surrogate parenting clinics under their direction. This was the case with Dr. Richard Levin's

Surrogate Parenting Associates in Louisville, Kentucky, and William W. Handel's Center of Surrogate Parenting in Beverly Hills, to give two examples.

Of the surrogate parenting clinics surveyed for this book, the largest worked with between 100 and 400 couples a year. A slightly larger roster of surrogates mothers was maintained to ensure availability. Among the clinics in this category were Dr. Levin's Surrogate Parenting Associates in Louisville, Kentucky, Noel Keane's Michigan operation and his Infertility Center of New York, and Harriet Blankfield's Infertility Associates in Chevy Chase, Maryland.

There was also a middle level of surrogate parenting clinics that handled twenty to forty cases a year. Representatives of these clinics included William Handel's Center of Surrogate Parenting and the Hagar Institute. Both centers claimed to offer individualized service. However, the majority of clinics surveyed operated on a small, intimate level, handling between five and twenty couples each year. People like Bernard Sherwyn, a Los Angeles lawyer, Kathryn Wyckoff of Reproductive Alternatives in San Clemente, California, Katie Brophy, a Louisville, Kentucky attorney and director of Surrogate Family Services, and Laraine Shore-Suslowitz, the director of the New England Surrogate Parenting Program in Springfield, Massachusetts, were operating one or two-person offices at the time they were contacted for the research on this book.

Bernard Sherwyn very much reflected the views of directors who have purposely kept their clinics small when he said he aims for warmth and personalized service. Sherwyn and his former partner, William Handel, were the first to open a surrogate parenting clinic in California. After a couple of years he left Handel's center and opened up his own law office and surrogate parenting center. For Sherwyn, the personal touch is what counts. "I like to know what's going on and keep personal contact. When you only have ten clients at a time you can be selective, and I find that I've put together a warm operation with a good feeling," he said. "I send people who want it businesslike to others [surrogate parenting centers]."

No surrogate parenting center, regardless of the client volume, was found to operate with more than seven full-time employees in the mid-1980s. The Center of Surrogate Parenting in Beverly Hills was the only one that reported working with a publicist. While some clinics relied on newspaper stories and word-of-mouth referrals to attract new business, at least nine clinics advertised regularly in local papers or nationwide. Only one clinic—Surrogate Parenting Associates in Louisville—reportedly did no advertising whatsoever.

Clinic directors have been able to maintain such small staffs by relying heavily on outside specialists—physicians, psychologists, lawyers, and social workers—to handle many aspects of their business. All of the clinics surveyed regularly referred surrogates and couples to professionals for at least one aspect of their operation—whether it was for artificial inseminations, legal work, or psychological screening. Sometimes the cost of outside work was included on the clinic's fee; at other times couples had to pay the outside professionals separately.

In the absence of any state or nationwide standards for operating a surrogate parenting clinic or center, clinic directors have had to develop standards of their own. Oftentimes they have developed contracts and policies with the knowledge—which most passed on to their clients—that much of what they have stipulated may not be upheld in a court of law. Yet despite the lack of formalized clinic network or association or any standardized means of communications, clinics across the country have exhibited surprising uniformity in their basic operating procedures. All of the clinics and centers surveyed for this book, with only one or two exceptions, screened both prospective couples and surrogates and charged fees for both their own and the surrogates' services. All clinics serviced only verifiably infertile couples. And all of them guided the artificial insemination process, assisted both parties during the pregnancy, and made arrangements for the birth. Some clinics offered counseling on the adoption procedure, however none got involved in the actual legal process.

Where the surrogate parenting centers and clinics surveyed tended to differ was in atmosphere and attitude. In some cases the directors and owners reflected the attitudes of the region in which they operate. West Coast directors, for instance, seemed a bit more open, more psychologically oriented, and less concerned with social form than did their eastern and midwestern colleagues. Some California clinics were especially publicity-conscious, working hard through their surrogates and couples to paint a positive picture of surrogate parenting in the wake of negative press stirred up by the "Baby M" custody battle. Clinic directors on the West Coast also talked more about personal fulfillment and serving others than about profit, while some midwestern and East Coast directors spoke openly about surrogate parenting as a business.

The personal attitudes of its owners and directors can greatly influence a clinic's operating procedures. For example, the survey conducted for this book revealed clinics that favor anonymity between couples and surrogates and those that insist on contact. This is why those interested in surrogate parenting should shop around before choosing a clinic. (See the Appendix for specifics on clinics in the United States.) Questioning owners or managers about personal styles and attitudes is crucial to selecting a program that will fulfill one's expectations. Many of the complaints of individuals interviewed for this book centered around differences in style between a couple or surrogate and the clinic. But for the most part these were complaints and problems that might have been avoided if those involved had examined themselves and their own styles first and then set about finding a clinic with similar attitudes about important issues such as anonymity, cost, and service.

As discussed throughout this book, one of the most difficult issues both couples and surrogates must come to terms with is that of determining how much contact their relationship should involve. Because attitudes and approaches to anonymity differ widely from one clinic to another, both prospective surrogates and couples should be careful to select a surrogate parenting clinic or center that matches their assessment of the kind of relationship they would like to establish. All prospective couples or surrogates who approach a surrogate parenting clinic or center are required to go through some kind of interview and/or screening process at the outset. Most clinics require both the couple and the surrogate to pass a physical and psychological exam. However, the nature of the screening differed from one clinic to another. Some surrogate parenting operations required genetic studies; others looked for criminal tendencies; and tests for Herpes and AIDS were becoming more common when research for this book was done. Although no clinic reported checking criminal records, most directors agreed that even a hint of a criminal past usually disqualified a couple or a surrogate from participation in their program. Beth Bacon, the director of the surrogate parenting program at the Hagar Institute, summarized the views of other clinic directors on this score when she said, "Everyone should have a second chance, but not in my program." The director of a West Coast surrogate parenting center added, "If I even had a question of a criminal past, I wouldn't accept them in the first place."

Many clinic directors were equally wary of couples and surrogate mothers who appear to be desperate for the procedure, or parties that seem to have been coerced into going along with this means of having a child. To weed out these potential problems, prospective clients—both couples and surrogates—were not only tested initially but sent on to a social worker or psychologist for further testing. And, as described earlier, many California clinics regularly provided group therapy sessions for couples and surrogates.

At Wyckoff's clinic, Reproductive Alternatives, both couples and surrogates were subjected to lengthy interviews before being sent on to a psychologist, a physician, or a lawyer. Candidates could be eliminated from the program at any time during this procedure if they did not meet with Wyckoff's approval or that of the other consulting professionals. She was especially concerned that her couples be emotionally ready for the commitment they had made: "If anything goes wrong, I don't want to be the cause of destroying a marriage," she said. "I make sure they understand the risks."

Psychologists in the field are divided on whether this kind of screening is adequate. Many made their concerns public during the course of the "Baby M" custody battle. During the trial Philip Parker—the Detroit psychologist who has conducted screenings for Keane's clinic—argued that no test had been devised that could determine whether a surrogate would actually relinquish her child. In the absence of such a test, he explained that he passed on any willing candidates for surrogacy who approached Keane's clinic. Other experts who testified in court during the "Baby M" custody battle argued that the psychological screening administered by Keane's clinic amounted to no screening at all. They feel there should be some means of determining whether the surrogate mother will be willing to relinquish the child after birth.

While no one has defended Keane in this instance, other clinic directors nationwide have agreed that there is a lack of hard, clinical data defining the components of proper screening. And in the absence of such data they vociferously defend their individual screening processes, no matter how cursory the process appears to be. Some, especially those with training in psychology or social work, said they base a

lot of their decisions on "intuition" and "trust." They pointed to the absence of any serious problems with either surrogates or couples in their programs as proof of the efficacy of
their screening methods.

"I think the key to screening is really face-to-face contact—spending enough time to get a feeling for the surrogate," Sherwyn said. "There's a lot of intuition involved.
You need to be a good judge of character. A problem is the
last thing you want. It's better to go through ten to twenty
than to have one [problem]." Harriet Blankfield, who insists
on extensive screening at Infertility Associates—everything
from AIDS, Herpes, Hepatitis B, and a sperm analysis for the
father to complete medical checks for both members of the
couple, an infertility test for the adoptive mother, and medical and psychological tests for couples and surrogates—
feels that all this testing is more than good business. "The
by-product of the process is an innocent child," she explained. "The crux of responsibility lies with the couple.
How can you overlook that?"

As thoroughly as clinic directors appeared to examine
prospective clients for possible medical and psychological
problems, only one or two of those surveyed seemed to conduct any extensive financial screening. Some form of financial statement from couples and surrogates was generally required at clinics nationwide. Clinic directors reported
checking for credit-card debts, and most of them did not accept women who were on welfare as surrogate mothers.
This was reported by many directors to be one of the safe-
guards against accepting women whose main motive for offering their services is the money. As for couples, they were
usually required to pay their clinic fee up front. The fee was
often held in an escrow account until the birth of the child.

Because of the nature of the fees—clinic charges ranged
from $4,000 to $12,000 nationwide at the time of writing
and surrogate fees from $8,500 to $12,000 plus expenses—
many clinic directors agreed that credit checks for couples

were unnecessary. They said the fees themselves served as a screening device. It is interesting to note the uniformity of surrogate fees despite the lack of any nationwide standardization of the fee structure. Ten out of eleven clinics surveyed chose $10,000 as the baseline fee for the surrogate mother, with half of these acknowledging additional expenses. Clinic fees were more varied, though a majority of the clinics surveyed charged between $9,000 and $12,000. The single exception was a West Coast director who has been waging a personal battle to keep fees accessible to many people. Aware of what she considers to be exorbitant fees being charged elsewhere, this person—who requested anonymity—has set her fee at $6,000 to prevent surrogate parenting from "becoming a business."

As a result of complaints from many couples about open-ended contracts that have forced them to pay a variety of unexpected expenses, about half of the clinics surveyed now have the couple and surrogate negotiate a detailed contract up front. In all of these cases, the surrogates and the couples agreed on everything from medical expenses to health insurance and day-care costs. Exactly how long after the birth the surrogate's expenses are expected to be covered is also negotiated. At least one clinic specified in its contract that couples are responsible for birth-related medical expenses—and only birth-related medical expenses—for two months postpartum. The remainder of the clinics surveyed were less specific and required couples to pick up postpartum medical expenses for an unspecified time. Despite the lack of detail in some contracts, most clinic directors seemed to feel it was unfair to have couples cover surrogate expenses indefinitely. "You can't financially bond a surrogate to the couple for life," explained Blankfield.

Once a couple has chosen a clinic and has agreed to the fees involved, they then face the issue of how to impregnate a strange woman. Artificial insemination procedures can differ widely from clinic to clinic and center to center. Two of the clinics surveyed refused to work with anything but fresh semen because they felt this would minimize the chances of a mix-up in paternity. At these two clinics the place of insemination was predetermined and the prospective father was required to produce a fresh sample at that location. Although this has been an effective way of safeguarding paternity, requiring fresh sperm samples can involve a great deal of travel and expense for the couple—especially since the effort must often be repeated many times before the surrogate mother becomes pregnant.

A Washington state couple reported that they had to pay a physician $300 for each insemination attempt, resulting in a total outlay of $1,200 before the surrogate mother became pregnant. For this reason most surrogate parenting clinics in this country allow their clients to use either fresh or frozen semen. Because frozen semen can be shipped, the actual insemination can take place anywhere. Clinics that used frozen semen usually allowed the surrogate mother to select the time and location of insemination. Two or three of them required the surrogate to use the physician affiliated with the clinic, which meant she had to do some traveling. In some cases, however, the couple and the surrogate agreed on a mutually convenient insemination site.

Whether or not surrogates and couples negotiated through a third party or worked directly very much depended on the clinic they had chosen. Clinic directors nationwide are roughly divided between those who think contact is not only desirable but makes for a healthier outcome and those who are adamantly opposed to any contact between couples and their surrogates. When it comes to anonymity, there appears to be very little middle ground. "Total anonymity, complete and forever," advocated Blankfield. "If you don't develop a relationship, you have none to terminate. I think getting to know each other is a bad policy. If a surrogate and a couple are very much desirous of this, I tell them to go to another agency." She added that she felt a child "deserved one father and one mother; otherwise you're confusing the child." The director of a West Coast center said, "I feel that establishing any permanent relationship is asking for future problems." It's more comfortable for the surrogate mother to make a clean break, and that's best done by maintaining anonymity. There's no reason for contact."

Other directors felt just as strongly that contact between surrogates and couples made for a far more pleasant, more meaningful pregnancy and birth. They saw no problems with couples and surrogates maintaining contact if they chose to do so. Neither did they think it was necessarily awkward for the surrogate to become involved in the child's life. In the wake of the "Baby M" case, Wyckoff argued that it's more important than ever for couples and surrogate mothers to meet and develop a relationship of trust. In cases where the surrogate remained an unknown, she said, the couple generally was terrified of her. "They're sure she'll take the child back at some time. I can't tell you how many calls I've had [from couples] because of that fear," she explained. It has been her experience that the fear subsides once the couple and the surrogate meet and discover that they're "real human beings." She added, "When people meet and look each other in the eye and talk about what's important to them, it's less likely the surrogate will want to keep the child."

At William Handel's Center of Surrogate Parenting, according to Hanafin, contact between all parties is actively encouraged. In fact, couples and surrogates meet and must choose to work together. The consensus here is that anonymity isn't beneficial. "We want surrogates and couples to know each other as a means of easing the separation process," Hanafin explained. The Hagar Institute has worked out something of a compromise on the anonymity issue. According to Bacon, both couples and surrogates are given one another's first names and—with the assistance of the institute—encouraged to exchange letters during the pregnancy.

They are allowed to meet at the hospital after the birth—a system she says "works beautifully!"

Bacon instituted this partial anonymity policy after discovering—from surrogates and couples who came to the Hagar Institute after being discouraged by other surrogate parenting programs—that contact could be difficult for the infertile woman (adoptive mother)." It was hard on them to be confronted by the surrogates' problems," she explained. Some felt they were too involved. They had to hold the surrogate's hand while she was being inseminated. It made them feel a lot more stressed." Contact also proved to be a problem for the institute, she said. "We worried about them not liking each other during the pregnancy. We worried about relinquishment. At least the letter writing gives them access to each other. They get to know each other. It's close with just the right amount of distance." Sherwyn, who generally leaves the decision of whether a couple and surrogate get to know each other up to them, believes that some involvement is helpful. "It's more realistic to maintain contact. This is a contract situation, but a very intimate one," he said.

For the few clinics that have absolutely insisted on maintaining anonymity, problems can and have arisen once the surrogate mother has entered a hospital to deliver. Surrogates and couples who are trying to maintain anonymity have literally bumped into each other at nursery windows. In some states the names of all parties concerned appeared on the birth certificate.

Blankfield, who of all the clinic directors was most concerned about maintaining anonymity, has worked out a system for ensuring that neither the couples nor the surrogates learn one another's identity while in the hospital for the birth. First, all of her births take place in the vicinity of her Chevy Chase clinic. When the surrogate goes into labor, she contacts the couple and directs them to the hospital waiting room, the lobby, or the cafeteria. Following the birth, she or a nurse brings the baby—tagged with the parent's names—to them. According to Blankfield, the surrogate is then moved to a wing outside the nursery area "to spare her feelings and keep people from running into each other." But the baby is shown only to the parents after that. "The surrogate sees the child at the time she delivers. She definitely needs that moment, but that's it," said Blankfield. According to Blankfield these precautions were taken for the baby's sake. "The baby is taken to the nursery and to the parents to allow them to bond. The surrogate," she said, "has done the job. If she's the appropriate woman she won't have the need to hold the baby and bond."

When it is time to fill out the birth certificate, Blankfield said the hospital first sends the form to the surrogate mother. She circles her questions and then the form is sent to the father. Both forms are then brought to the medical records department, where a composite is made. The fact that the state of Maryland does not require a signature for either party makes it much easier to retain anonymity between couples and surrogate mothers, she said, adding, "With proper laws anonymity shouldn't be an issue."

Because the majority of clinics surveyed did not expend a great deal of effort in maintaining anonymity and even encouraged contact—including allowing couples to participate in the delivery room—the hospital was not a troublesome setting. In fact, clinic directors nationwide reported that the hospitals they work with are now invariably cooperative when it comes to surrogate births. Most hospitals appear to treat births by surrogacy very much like adoptions. (It must be noted, however, that there are hospitals and doctors—especially those affiliated with the Catholic church—that would not allow a surrogate birth if that fact were known.)

Although almost all of the recorded births by surrogate mother had produced healthy babies at the time of this writing, there is always the chance of a stillbirth or of a child being born with a birth defect. In 1983 there was a case in which a father refused to accept as his a child born with microcephaly (a small head, usually associated with retardation) and the surrogate mother said she felt no maternal bond to the child. As it turned out, a paternity test revealed that the man involved was not the father after all. The baby was the natural child of the surrogate and her husband. A flurry of suits and countersuits ensued.

In an attempt to avoid this and other related issues, all clinic directors surveyed for this book had formulated some kind of policy regarding stillbirths or babies born with birth defects. In the event of a stillbirth, at least six clinics required couples to pay the surrogate the agreed-upon expenses but not the fee if the pregnancy was not brought to term. Should the pregnancy go full-term the surrogate would receive her fee and the clinic would then allow the couple to impregnate another surrogate, in this case waiving the fee.

Some of the clinics surveyed allowed the surrogate partial payment of her fee if the baby were born dead and full payment if the child survived twenty-four hours or longer. In both instances, the clinic would then waive its fee and allow the couple to try again. At least one clinic would simply terminate the entire contract, including further payments to the surrogate mother, in the event of a stillbirth or defective birth. And two others handled this problem by having the parties involved negotiate their own resolution of the issue before artificial insemination took place.

Policies directed at resolving the issue of birth defects proved to be far more uniform nationwide than those concerning stillbirths. Nine clinics of the fifteen surveyed considered the baby to be the couple's responsibility regardless of its physical or mental condition. Two of the clinics surveyed allowed both couple and surrogate to negotiate this point prior to artificial insemination.

Despite the criticism of questionable screening processes and the lack of uniform policies and laws to guide clinic directors, surrogate parenting has led a relatively trouble-free existence. For the most part surrogates have been impregnated, carried the fetus to term, and willingly relinquished healthy babies to happy parents. As of this writing, the "Baby M" case was the only well-publicized incident of a surrogate refusing to give up a child. Clinic directors reported that any breach of contract they experienced took place before artificial insemination.

Given the diversity of political and religious beliefs represented in this country—the Catholic church and Orthodox Jews have condemned the practice—it's interesting to note that few clinics reported having problems with either their state governments or conservative political or religious groups. The notable exceptions have been in Michigan, Kentucky, and Ohio. In an attempt to outlaw "baby buying" Michigan law has prohibited payment of money for an adoption. Noel Keane challenged the law with a test case in 1978. Denied throughout the Michigan court system, he eventually appealed to the U.S. Supreme Court, which ruled eight to one not to consider the case. According to Lori Andrews in *New Conceptions,* Keane has subsequently found ways to work within the law.

In 1981 the Kentucky attorney general attempted to shut down Surrogate Parenting Associates on grounds that the operation was practicing "baby buying." The clinic's right to operate was eventually upheld by the state supreme court, setting a legal precedent for other clinics in the state.

Wyckoff moved her Ohio surrogate parenting clinic to California in 1984 after the state attorney general threatened to arrest her on charges of soliciting women. According to Wyckoff, this was a scare tactic to force her to shut down her clinic. At a meeting between state officials and her attorney, the state agreed to drop charges if she would close up shop. Wyckoff told her attorney she wanted to fight. In fact, she was prepared to take out a second mortgage on her house to finance a legal battle when the attorney general was voted out of office.

Although the new attorney general did not pursue the

battle, Wyckoff decided to take her practice to a more conge-
nial climate. However, she is adamant on the point that she
was willing to fight if that proved necessary. As an infertile
woman who plans to have her own child with the assistance
of a surrogate mother, Wyckoff can be said to have a very
personal stake in the concept of surrogate parenting. "I truly
believe women can have babies for other people," she said.
"I've met many infertile couples and my heart aches for
them."

As of this writing, Kansas was the only state that recognized surrogate parenting clinics and required them to be licensed. Arkansas is the only state with a law on the books
making surrogate parenting legal and recognizing the adoptive mother as the child's legal guardian. Beth Bacon, the director of the Hagar Institute, in Topeka, Kansas, has found
state officials "helpful and friendly," and the backing of the
law useful for the clinic's reputation. "They realize we're
not a bunch of weirdos. We're social workers who want to
work according to good medical and psychological practices," she said.

Although almost all surrogate parenting cases to date
have ended happily, many clinic directors have conceded
that they've been lucky. In most areas of the country the law
is on the natural mother's side. Every director or owner of a
surrogate parenting clinic interviewed realized that they
could be the next to be hit with a sensational custody case.
At the time of the "Baby M" case, Keane—whose clinic
united the Sterns and Whitehead—told a number of publi-
cations that the New Jersey custody battle "was a case waiting to happen, somewhere, sometime." He added, "Nobody can tell you today what somebody is going to do nine
months from now."

Other Clinic directors tended to underplay the potential
for a "Baby M" case at their clinic, with their clients. Blankfield might have been speaking for all of her colleagues
when she said the New Jersey Whitehead-Stern case would
never have happened if proper protocol had been observed.

But she added, "Still, there but for the grace of God go I."

She and Hanafin agreed that working with the surrogate mother and helping her with relinquishing the child can go a long way to staving off a situation in which the surrogate finds it impossible to give up the baby. While Hanafin has set up a well-publicized group counseling program for surrogates, Blankfield requires the women she employs to see a psychologist for at least six months following the birth. Since instituting this policy, she reported that she has seen very little postpartum depression. "Most surrogates don't feel the child is theirs," she explained. "They feel they're carrying it for someone else and can detach themselves from the child. They really want to see the wellness of the child, but nothing more."

In the interest of the surrogate mother and the couple, most of the clinics surveyed reported maintaining some sort of contact with both parties indefinitely. However, clinic directors have noted that they hear more from surrogates than from couples. Couples usually drift away several months after the birth to resume their lives. The majority of clinics reported making an effort to stay in almost daily contact with the surrogate mother for a month after birth and then slackening the contact over the period of a year.

Opponents of surrogate parenting—particularly fertility experts in the United States and Great Britain—have expressed concern about the monetary aspects of the process. They question whether either a middleman or the surrogate mother should receive financial remuneration for their services. Some of the medical experts involved in drafting the Wornak report have suggested that if surrogate parenting clinics or centers are allowed to exist at all, they should operate on a nonprofit basis.

That suggestion has met with a resounding no from all clinic directors surveyed for this book. Some have argued that it makes little difference whether their clinics operate on a nonprofit basis because money will still change hands, and they will still earn a salary. In that case, they have maintained, it makes no sense to bar the profit motive in some vain effort to purify surrogate parenting. Other directors have found the suggestion unfeasible because of the large quantities of time-consuming paperwork involved with a non-profit organization, and the remaining clinic directors simply said they worked hard and deserved some reward for their services.

"I'm a capitalist and I believe in it," Sherwyn said. "I feel services are better performed by someone who benefits by doing them. If you compare almost any service done in a nonprofit way with those done in a profit setting, you're going to find that there's a more personalized and humane approach in the profit setting." He also added, "Most clinics want the thing to work out. I was born in L. A., I work here and have a legal license to protect. I'm not about to conduct a fly-by-night business."

A number of clinic directors laughed at the suggestion that they should assume a nonprofit status when they haven't yet realized a profit from their business. "We are for profit, but we haven't made much," Bacon said of the Hagar Institute. "In 1985 it was 2 percent and in 1986 we may not have a profit." If run correctly, Blankfield feels that surrogate parenting centers will show no profit at the end of the year. "It costs a lot of money to provide this service," she said. "We have telephone bills of $1,500 a month because it's important to keep in touch [with clients]. I'm paid a salary as director along with the other staff."

Noel Keane, who is considered by some to be the founder of the business because he opened the first known surrogate parenting clinic in 1976, said the money issue is "a red herring for religious discontent for what we [the clinics and centers] are doing." He added, "If you took away the money issue, you would find the same people objecting to the issue [surrogate parenting]." According to Keane, the middleman or clinic director is essential to the process. Clinic directors, he said, both attract and screen surrogates. And for this effort Keane feels they should be paid. He knows that he has engendered much resentment as a lawyer "earning a substantial amount of money off infertility," but he has argued that it is necessary. "It isn't impure. There's nothing wrong with it. I'm giving professional services and so is the surrogate," he said. In fact, Keane has estimated that based on a $10,000 fee, the average surrogate mother will net $6,000 after taxes. "Divide that by the hours [of her service from insemination attempts to birth] and she will probably earn sixty to seventy-nine cents an hour for the risk of facing bleeding or even death," he said.

If they are united on the financial issue, clinic directors have been somewhat divided on whether to allow some form of standardization or regulation of the procedure on either a state or national basis. All of those interviewed for this book agreed that legalization of surrogate parenting is necessary, and the majority felt that some standards would be helpful, including standards governing clinic directors themselves. But several clinic directors have said they were wary of government intervention into or even a downright ban of their business. Half of those surveyed, however, thought regulation would be necessary if the procedure is to become uniformly reliable and respected. A West Coast director summed up the position of those who are leery: "Some legislation is definitely needed, but regulation by the government does not sound appealing."

In Massachusetts, Laraine Shore-Suslowitz has spoken in favor of standardization of services and some controls on operating procedures but has opposed government regulation. Another West Coast director supported the government "designing and creating some sort of criteria" as long as mounds of time-consuming paperwork would not be created along with the standards. Blankfield, too, favors regulation if regulation does not equal censorship. "I do feel there should be legislation and rules," she affirmed. According to Blankfield the first law would be a national or state-by-state move to legalize surrogate parenting. The second would be a law recognizing the adoptive mother as the legal mother, which would obviate the need for the adoption process and eliminate custody battles.

She has also recommended institution of a number of standards, including the requirement that the couple be certifiably infertile and that a woman serve as a surrogate only once. With the enactment of these rules, Blankfield said she hoped to prevent creation of a "a breeder class" among surrogates. "The only reason a woman would want to participate as a surrogate repeatedly is for money," she explained. "I want to limit this to one time. I believe altruism falls by the wayside by the third time. On paper it's nice to have one surrogate create two children for a family, but it's a double tie. Twenty years down the line you're going to see a problem with the children."

Finally, Blankfield suggested that a psychological and medical evaluation be mandatory for all participants in the process. And she believes the evaluations should be conducted by referral to avoid the problem of the clinics turning these procedures into profit-making ventures. As for fees, she has advocated that they be uniform nationwide and be set high enough to cover expenses but not so high as to give anyone a windfall: "We keep telling everyone we're not selling babies; it's a service. But you put it in that category when you start bartering. I want to see surrogacy in a pure form—not haggling."

Hanafin and Bacon were also extremely supportive of licensing surrogate parenting operations and standardizing procedures. According to Hanafin, the Beverly Hills clinic and its director, William Handel, have actively lobbied the California legislature in an attempt to gain support and guidance for surrogate parenting clinics in California. Their main concern, she said, is preventing abuse by creating legislation that would outline the proper way of operating a clinic. As of this writing, the California legislature had tabled all such attempts.

As director of the only clinic that is reported to be operating under state licensure, Bacon spoke from experience on this matter. (Arkansas has a law on the books recognizing surrogate parenting and making the adoptive mother the legal parent, but no known clinics existed there at the time of this writing.) To keep standards high, she believes some regulation is needed. And she agreed with other clinic directors who support change in the laws to facilitate recognition of who's entitled to and responsible for the child: "The laws should include a requirement that legal representation be provided the surrogate, and they should outline the sort of screening conducted." Bacon added that some kind of counseling should be required for both the couple and the surrogate mother.

Wyckoff also supported regulation and control of some nature: "You can't dictate morality, but I feel there should be some way to keep people on the straight and narrow. A way of pulling a license if something unethical were done." She was not alone in her fear that anyone—at the time of this writing—could establish a surrogate parenting clinic or center. For Wyckoff, instituting some controls on the process are equal to "protecting surrogate parenting."

As an attorney, Sherwyn feels it will makes things a lot easier if the government recognizes surrogate parenting and makes his contracts binding. However, he said legalization isn't the entire key to making the process more workable. And as much as he favors changing the law to recognize the adoptive mother as the legal mother from the point of conception, he did not feel that was the key either: "I feel the key is getting to know the couples and surrogates more than passing legislation. Even if the adoptive mother was made the legal mother before birth, no hospital would let the baby out of its jurisdiction without the birth mother's authorization." Sherwyn has warned that any legal changes will be slow and will be won on a state-by-state basis. The federal government, he said, will not handle issues surrounding family and fertility.

Although the laws may be stacked against them and their procedural styles are essentially individualistic, all of the surrogate parenting directors interviewed argued that their services are much needed. Moreover, they argued that they are doing a good job. As proof they pointed to the number of people who call them on a weekly basis and the number of cases that were successfully completed by the winter of 1987. "I've been doing this for five years and I see people coming back a second and a third time. For me, that's the greatest compliment," Wyckoff said. "No one would return if they hadn't had a positive, good experience."

Clinic directors also pointed to the diversity of clinics as a sign of the strength of the surrogacy movement. "One of the good things about this country is that we have options," Blankfield said. "There are enough agencies to allow you to shop for comparisons; go where you think it's going to be more comfortable and things will be handled best."

According to Sherwyn, "The key is treating people like people; the way you'd like to be treated. Things run most smoothly when you're not trying to manipulate people." He has always tried to create a situation in which attitudes between couples and surrogates gel: "I want them doing it out of desire, not fear." Bacon added, "There are hassles, fears and risks, but overall, people really do get a baby. I feel it's extremely worthwhile. Society should take this process seriously," she said, "and we'll keep on protecting it."

# 4
## MORAL AND ETHICAL ISSUES

# 9 | Unresolved Questions

Witnessing a newborn in the arms of its adoring adoptive parents, it is difficult to understand why the issue of surrogate parenting—or any of the "new" reproductive techniques, for that matter—should generate such a storm of protest. Thanks to these new reproductive technologies, infertile couples can now have children of their own. One wonders, isn't it the end result that counts?

Sometimes, but not always. For as much as we like to see infertile couples able to have children, there's much more to surrogate parenting than the end result. Surrogacy is an emotionally complicated process that involves many players. Couples have family and friends who become involved in the surrogate birth. The surrogate mother often has a husband or a boyfriend and children who must cope with her actions. And then there is the child—a child who must someday assimilate the knowledge that he or she was created with the assistance of an unknown third party. And, more disturbing in some cases, that someone paid a price for his or her birth.

There are so many people, so many potential interpersonal problems, that it's little wonder that while most of us approve of the end result of surrogate parenting—creating a child for infertile couples—just as many privately admit that the process makes them uneasy. Philosophers and experts in applied ethics say this is because the procedure raises a variety of questions that challenge traditional values surrounding motherhood, love, procreation, parenthood, and the use of one's body for profit.

One of these people who have probed the moral and ethical implications of the new reproductive techniques is Arthur Caplan, a leading expert in applied ethics. Caplan, who until June 1987 served as associate director of the Hastings Center, Hastings-on-Hudson, New York, is currently director of the Biomedical Ethics Center at the University of Minnesota.

As of this writing Caplan had written an article on the ethics of in vitro fertilization and agreed to talk about the ethics of surrogate parenting for this book. Although he considers it his job to question the impact of the new reproductive techniques on society—including surrogate parenting, artificial insemination, microsurgery, fertility drugs, and various forms of in vitro fertilization—Caplan is not antagonistic to these procedures. However, he is concerned with the effect they can have on basic social institutions such as the family, kinship, and parenting, as well as on society at large. Consequently, he has advocated that some form of control be placed on their use.

At the time of this interview Caplan was still sorting out his feelings about many of the new reproductive techniques. In principle, he said, he is not against surrogate parenting. In this procedure, Caplan feels, it is at least "possible for someone to give consent, voluntarily and freely, to carry someone's sperm or sperm and egg [embryo transfer]. There are many worse ways to earn a living and we let people do them every day," he pointed out. "Mining, for example, or work in high construction or on an assembly plant—many are riskier and tougher jobs [than being a surrogate mother]."

Whatever our feelings about surrogate parenting and the other new forms of reproductive technology, Caplan has argued that society should accept that these procedures are here to stay, and should allow them to be brought into the mainstream by licensing and standardizing them. He has contended that with the number of private arrangements already taking place, an outright ban of something like surrogate parenting can only drive the process underground. That is precisely what has happened with prostitution and prohibition, he said.

While Caplan considers outlawing these procedures to be useless, he is troubled by the fact that society has not moved to legalize and subsequently control the practice of the new reproductive technologies. By turning its head, he feels that society is allowing these practices to grow and flourish in a climate that may not only be detrimental to some but may change how society itself allocates its resources. For example, he argued that increased demand for the means of alleviating infertility, coupled with increased usage of experimental procedures, will only require additional allocation of resources in this direction. An increase that "raises profoundly disturbing and complex moral issues." ("The Ethics of In Vitro Fertilization," *Biomedical Ethics*, June 1986.)

Much of Caplan's moral/ethical analysis of in vitro fertilization can be applied to the issue of surrogate parenting. Of special interest is his concern that the new generation of infertility interventions may create "basic moral issues" surrounding "informed consent, liability for untoward results, and public policies concerning reimbursement." One of his primary questions is whether infertility is a disease that requires medical intervention. To treat infertility as such, Caplan said, raises additional questions. These are largely questions of equity and justice that fall roughly into two broad categories—social justice and individual justice. Problems created by various treatments for infertility become matters of public concern, according to Caplan, if society has to pick and choose how to allocate funds for combating disease. As of 1986, he estimated that $200 million was being spent annually to fight infertility. He has predicted that there will be future funding conflicts if increased demand for technologically based services are coupled with continued health-care funding cuts. But the question of how to fund these procedures pales next to the issue of whether infertile couples should be creating babies through extraordinary means at a time when many "undesirable" children—especially the physically or mentally handicapped—can't find adoptive parents. And, Caplan questions, should any of these procedures exist side-by-side with abortion?

In terms of individual justice, Caplan is concerned with the cost of the new reproductive technologies. Some, he feels, are prohibitively expensive, which effectively restricts their use "to those who can pay for them, either out of pocket, or in some cases through private insurance." He pointed out that geography and access to information also limit the number of people who can take advantage of these procedures.

If society is to sort out these and other issues that may arise from the new technologies of reproduction, Caplan has suggested that it must first come to terms with its underlying distaste for any procedures that deviate from centuries-old attitudes. "Attitudes about conception, child rearing and the nature of the family," he said, "are greatly influenced by social and ethical beliefs concerning individual rights, the duties of marriage, and the desirability of passing a particular set of genetic information on to the next generation." (*Biomedical Ethics*, June 1986.)

According to Caplan, any tampering with these attitudes creates inner conflicts that in turn make us feel uncomfortable about taking advantage of the new techniques for alleviating infertility. For example, our belief that people should have a right to do whatever they choose with their own bodies may be in conflict with an aversion to using the body for profit—taking something that is based on the sanctity of life and commercializing it. Surrogate parenting, he feels, can also turn motives upside down, creating a sea of moral confusion. Caplan and others in his field have argued that motives have a great deal to do with whether the outcome of a procedure such as surrogate parenting is deemed morally acceptable. When something as positive as the creation of a child is mixed with less than pure motives—financial gain, for example—the result can be public outcry.

This, to a large extent, is what has occurred with surrogate parenting. While no one deplores helping infertile couples have a baby, many question the motives of those involved in the process. Some question whether the couples, the surrogate mothers, and the clinic directors are working for long-term good or for personal gain. With the introduction of the new reproductive technologies, Caplan believes the motives for procreation have become increasingly skewed. Love, for example, has historically been the primary motivation behind natural pregnancy. With a procedure such as surrogate parenting, however, that may no longer be the case. According to Caplan, the biological mother may act "out of self-interest for something commercial, which seems strange or even upsetting to a lot of people." Caplan added, "So if you take motives seriously, what you now have is the change of pregnancy from something that normally was motivated by virtue to something that isn't a virtue and isn't quite a vice. This makes it unsettling; not quite right."

There are other possible underlying motives in surrogate parenting that don't feel quite right. The profit motive is one of them. While it is generally conceded that surrogate mothers and clinic directors should be compensated for their work, the inclusion of money is what many people have found unsettling. According to Caplan, this is because in Judeo-Christian thinking, "it's better to act from charity and love than from profit." He added, "I agree. I generally think love and charity are better motives than profit." Symbolically, he said, money has the "psychological implication of making things cheap and dirty." Babies, on the other hand, are perceived as pure. "This is one of the reasons there's something strange to us about mixing motherhood and money," said Caplan. "It's more a cultural association than an ethical one. Only women can be mothers, and mothers, in turn, are considered to be special. Mothers are ideally seen as pure creatures who do things relative to children out of love. Money has no such idealistic connotations."

Furthermore, he feels that most people are uncomfortable with the idea of placing a monetary value on human life. According to Caplan, birth is one area that hasn't seen much commercialization because "we try to think of life as priceless." He added, "When you do pay a large sum for a child, $25,000 for example, that does put a price on that child." Should this practice become more acceptable, Caplan has predicted that society will see further commercialization of birth—"motherhood up in neon lights." And with that, commercialization will have encroached on just about every aspect of our society. But not, Caplan feels, without further debate over such questions as whether there is any proper use of the body for commercial gain and whether it is proper to allow people to put themselves at physical risk. Even those who support free use of the body for whatever purpose the individual desires stop short of activities that put someone "at risk of death," according to Caplan. "And pregnancy," he said, "the centerpiece of surrogate parenting, does have some risk of that."

Other problems that can be demeaning ensue from selling one's body or its capacities. "For instance," he said, "people would feel devastated if they were forced to sell their blood to survive. Self-respect is crucial to freedom and dignity, which is why there are arguments against prostitution."

Whether those practices strike some as discomforting or improper, whether those involved in surrogate parenting are acting out of good or bad motives, the fact is that since 1980 thousands of infertile couples have hired surrogate mothers to bear their husbands' children. Rather than outlaw surrogate parenting, Caplan has come up with a number of recommendations he feels would help ensure that no one is hurt by the process.

First, he has suggested that the procedure be "standardized and regulated so that those involved understand the implications of their actions and can be guided throughout the process." Part of the problem with regulating surrogate parenting at this time, he said, is that it falls into the experimental category of procedures, along with in vitro fertilization and embryo transplant. He feels that society cannot easily regulate or even standardize "experimental processes that are supposed to be therapeutic."

Although clinic directors nationwide would differ with him, Caplan considers surrogate parenting to be experimental because many people are using the process without understanding its emotional, moral, or ethical implications. For this reason he has recommended that standards and regulations for surrogate parenting be implemented as soon as possible so that the marketplace does not serve as the only control. "It's terrible that anyone can open up a fertility clinic and go into business with only the market to regulate them," he said. "People have a right to informed consent."

Among the regulations Caplan has recommended is that surrogate parenting never be allowed for "convenience sake"—that women not be allowed to hire a surrogate mother simply because they do not have the time or inclination to bear their own children. To that end he had suggested that before they are being allowed to hire a surrogate mother, all adoptive mothers should be screened for infertility no matter how cumbersome the process might be. (In fact, all surrogate parenting clinics or centers interviewed for this book had a policy restricting their programs to truly infertile couples. Most of them required some form of proof from the couple.)

Caplan also suggested screening surrogate mothers because of the "biological uncertainty" they create. Most surrogate parenting clinics currently conduct some psychological, medical, and genetic testing of prospective surrogate mothers, but no standardized testing exists. Caplan has predicted that problems will issue from this vacuum of standards because there is no means of restricting surrogates in selling their services or of holding them accountable for these services. "Yet," he said, "we do this in other areas, such as sperm and blood banks, where you can sue for a bad product."

Many clinic directors have said that the price of the procedure serves as a screening process, at least for the couples. Caplan has agreed that price, or the market, is an effective if not equitable screening mechanism. However, he does not believe the price should be made so expensive that only the rich can afford the procedure. He also worries that by making a process such as surrogate parenting extremely expensive, hence lucrative, resources will be diverted from other health systems and health-care personnel will shift to the new reproductive technologies because of the financial incentives. Which leads to the question of whether money should change hands at all in surrogate parenting. Caplan doesn't agree with those—especially the writers of the Wornak report—who have suggested that surrogate parenting clinics be made non-profit for the purpose of "having as little money involved as possible."

According to Caplan the British are passsionately opposed to mixing finances with procedures that involve value-of-life questions. More so than Americans, he pointed out, the British consider it wrong to place a value on life and won't even pay people to donate plasma, even though the donation may take them away from work for at least half a day. Rather than pay for the donation, Caplan has pointed out that the British import American plasma—a practice he considers to be hypocritical.

Despite his own distaste for the commercialization of the new reproductive technologies, Caplan doesn't forsee them existing in modern society without the exchange of money. "A significant proportion of the population will want the process [surrogacy] and will need women," he said. "To get it, people will have to use their bodies, and money will change hands."

Caplan is more concerned with the related issues that result from the introduction of money into the procedure than with the actual idea of people selling their bodies for money. He pointed out that people like athletes and dancers use their bodies for money as a matter of course. "Part of the issue with money is that it brings problems with it—the potential for extortion or reneging on contracts," he said. The fact that the legal system hasn't caught up with the reality that surrogate parenting is very much alive and thriving in America leaves all parties involved open to abuses, Caplan said. For this reason he has urged "modifying the law to make all the contracts clear, binding, up front and enforceable."

And he went one step further, arguing that society's notion of parenting will have to change in order to accommodate the new reproductive technologies. In fact, Caplan said that procedures such as surrogate parenting are already altering our notion of motherhood and parenthood. If the law is to reflect reality, he believes that the adoptive or "social" mother should take legal precedence "because she's doing the mothering," and she should take that legal precedence from the time a contract is signed. According to Caplan, the biological or "gestational" mother should be considered a person who "houses eggs."

In his *Biomedical Ethics* article, Caplan wrote that the courts and the government have been slow to respond because of a longtime disagreement over the proper role of the law and the state "in influencing or controlling individual decisions concerning reproduction." He added that "traditionally, American courts have been loath to countenance any interference with matters pertaining to the family and individual decisions concerning procreation."

Caplan also hopes that with the increased concern the courts are now showing for protecting the interests of newborns and children, society and the law will alter its views of parenthood and accept the rights of the adoptive parent as preeminent. He pointed out that other societies have very different attitudes about adoption—attitudes that are far less obsessional about the rights of the biological parents. However, he feels it is important for the child involved to know who its biological parent is, but primarily for medical reasons.

He has suggested that those who embrace a process such as surrogate parenting be mindful of how this procedure can "threaten the family if not treated with care." Caplan can't imagine anyone wanting to live in a family "that's together because someone paid enough to stick the family members in one household." He added, "I want a family with responsibilities to each other, not debts. I want a family based on ethics, not the profit motive." With legal recognition and regulation on the part of society, and education, a thoughtful approach to the process, and pure motives on the part of those participating in the procedure, Caplan expressed hope that a technique such as surrogate parenting could continue to be used successfully to alleviate infertility.

Unlike Caplan, there are many experts in the field who would like to see surrogacy banned but have accepted the fact that this is a practical impossibility. Their goal is to convince society that this practice is morally unacceptable—a practice that should be discouraged. Daniel Callahan, director of the Hastings Center, is one of the most resolute opponents of surrogate parenting in this country. Callahan has serious misgivings about a process "that is built on confusion" and creates "a cadre of women whose prime virtue is what we now take to be deep vice—the bearing of a child one does not want and is prepared not to love."

He can see no way out of this moral dilemma. Regulation of the procedure, he said, forces society "to introduce procedures with disturbing implications. Neither is banning the commercialization of surrogate parenting the answer, he feels. "There would still be the need to find women with the capacity thoroughly to dissociate and distance themselves from their own child. This is not a psychological trait we should want to foster, even in the name of altruism," he said.

After weighing the pros and cons of the issue, after discussing whether the ends in this case justify the means, Callahan's answer was "no." He has argued that infertility is not a disease that is crippling society, that we already have "too many children being born under less than desirable circumstances," and that to encourage surrogate parenting would simply be "tolerating still another mode of producing children that is less than desirable or optimal." He has rejected the notion that society must start redefining its concept of parentage to conform with the realities of the new reproductive technologies. Rather, he feels the centuries-old concept of a biological mother and father should be upheld and that society should not foster procedures such as surrogate parenting, which, he feels, are "courting confusion about parentage."

Callahan's only answer to the issue of surrogate parenting seems to be that society should "chill out" the procedure by fostering a culture that considers such a practice to be morally unacceptable. Although he has no illusions that this will put an end to the practice, he argued that "there's a big difference between having it exist in a supportive context as opposed to one that's discouraging." He added, "All sorts of terrible things go on in our society. That doesn't mean that we should approve of them. It's pretty clear that this is becoming much more popular, that people are setting up businesses. It's clear that 'Baby M' increased the interest. I would bet that legalization and regulation of surrogate parenting would help the clinics."

In the end Callahan was torn on the issue of whether to legalize and regulate surrogacy. On the one hand, he doesn't want to encourage surrogate parenting. But on the other, he hates to see individuals—especially the surrogate mother—suffer because of the absence of proper controls and regulations. "My personal view," he said, "is that if we have to have some regulation, I would prefer laws that discourage the practice rather than encourage it. I would like to see laws banning the fee and a duration of time after the birth in which the surrogate mother may change her mind. The baby would be held in some neutral territory."

Neither Callahan nor Caplan, with their differing views, pretended to have all the answers. Those who side with Caplan will agree that society must accept surrogate parenting and adapt to it, while those who agree with Callahan will work to make the practice morally unacceptable before its impact on society can be felt too deeply.

# Epilogue

Without the slightest hesitation Bernie McRobbie gleefully ripped open the clown-covered paper, revealing a red truck to the group of family and friends who had gathered in the McRobbies' sunlit den to celebrate his first birthday. With a chortle the little blond boy tossed away the toy and went on to the next brightly wrapped present in the pile.

Sitting on the floor beside Bernie were his parents. The smiles on Glenn's and Linda's face could have lit up the sky on a moonless night. As Linda watched carefully to make sure the baby put nothing into his mouth, Glenn demonstrated the operation of each toy. Bernie's screeches of delight mingled with the cheers and applause of his loved ones.

No one, least of all the McRobbies, could have anticipated this scene a year ago. On April 9, 1986 the McRobbies' main concern was whether Bernie's biological mother—the surrogate Helen—would release the infant into their custody. Everything went as planned in the hospital. And for the most part Bernie's first year of life was a joy for his parents. Although both McRobbies remained anxious until Bernie was formally adopted at the age of six months, Helen never contested parenthood. When the McRobbies appeared before the judge one warm, October day, he gave his approval of the adoption without question.

But there were problems. Some could be attributed to legal issues surrounding surrogate parenting, some to the usual first-time parental annoyances and anxieties, and some to just plain circumstances. For a variety of reasons Glenn decided to leave his job at the bank early in the fall. His adjustment to a new job unfortunately coincided with Linda's adjustment to motherhood, resulting in some marital friction. As a new mother living in an isolated country home away from friends and support, Linda found the change from working woman to full-time mother more difficult than she had expected. Besides worrying that Helen would reassert some claim on Bernie, she did not always find Glenn supportive or helpful when it came to taking care of the baby. It surprised and annoyed her that he wasn't more involved in caring for the child he had fought for so long and so hard to have. Glenn, in turn, found Linda unsympathetic to the burdens of a new job, which left him little energy for Bernie at the end of the day.

Then, right after Thanksgiving, the unthinkable happened. Bernie woke one morning with what appeared to be a severe cold and was hospitalized that evening with a diagnosis of meningitis. Doctors told the McRobbies that their child was close to death at the time of his admittance to the hospital.

Although the hospital staff rallied behind the little boy, for several days Bernie—always a robust, active baby—was almost lifeless. For the next week either Glenn or Linda slept on a cramped cot by the baby's side. During this horrendous vigil Linda confided that Bernie's arrival had strained the marriage. She had resented her loss of freedom and Glenn's apparent lack of interest in a child he had so desperately wanted. But as she looked down at the jaundiced baby in the hospital crib, a little baby struggling for breath, she fought back the tears. "I don't know what I would do if died," she whispered. "He's become my whole life."

Bernie did recover, and within weeks was a bouncing, happy little boy again. The experience was a sobering one for Linda. Rather than give in to those feelings of despondency that had plagued her during the fall, she decided to expand her sphere of activity and took on part-time design work that she could do at home.

Glenn later admitted that he was aware of both Linda's feelings and the fact that surrogate parenting could breed resentment between a husband and wife. "I know Linda felt she sacrificed her biological role to give me a child, but I didn't have many choices," he explained. "I could either give up having a child altogether or have another woman bear the child." Glenn decided that it would be easier for Linda to sacrifice her role as biological mother than for their marriage to be childless. His father had advised him otherwise, but he had pooh-poohed the criticism. "I decided it was better that she resent me than that I resent her, and I'm glad I did it. Sure there was resentment in the air, sure we had to make some adjustments, but it was worth it. Linda's much happier now than she was when we were childless."

Certainly, as Bernie's first birthday approached and the snow drifts around the McRobbies' home shrank to puddles, Linda seemed a lot happier and much more secure in her new role. She and Glenn had decided to have another child, and they were actively seeking out a surrogate mother for what they hoped would be an embryo transfer this time, making Linda the biological mother.

If anything marred the McRobbies' happiness that spring it was the "Baby M" case. They received numerous requests from television stations and newspapers across the country

202 | S U R R O G A T E   P A R E N T I N G

to comment on the case. All the attention revived Linda's fears about Bernie's safety and Helen's intent, while Glenn found the media's focus on couples like themselves to be an excruciating replay of a very private pain. But at least this spring they had Bernie. All you had to do was call the McRobbies household and the first thing either Glenn or Linda would ask you was, "Do you hear Bernie laughing? Isn't he wonderful?" Yes, Bernie McRobbie was a wonderful, cheerful, happy, outgoing infant. The week before his first birthday, Glenn reported proudly, "Bernie's standing on his own."

As 1986 turned into 1987, Jane Woodman had little time to dwell on the few memories she had of the baby girl she had carried and given up to another couple. "Last summer I fantasized a lot about the baby, but since then I've been too busy working. That's all I've had time to do," she said. Once, when she was in the Boston area, she gave in to the urge to drive by the street where the baby now lives. "I did it out of curiosity," she said. The house was large and impressive. Jane drove on, feeling slightly saddened but relieved to see that the child she had produced for others would not want for anything materially.

Though fatiguing, Jane's job as a nurse in a maternity ward has proved extremely rewarding. After her first two pregnancies, she had feared assisting other women in labor. But she discovered that their experiences brought to mind her "successful" third delivery—the delivery as a surrogate mother. One of her big thrills that first year after the baby's birth was the picture she received at Christmas. "She really looks like she could be one of my kids and a sister of my kids. I was just thrilled," she gushed. "I even found myself showing close friends the picture."

Along with the picture came a nice letter from the family. There was only one disconcerting note. The couple wondered whether Jane would be willing to act as a surrogate mother for them again. The request was tempting, but at thirty-eight Jane felt she was too old to get pregnant for someone else. "It would be too tiring. Anyway," she added, "the one goal I haven't accomplished is to have another baby for my family. I still cherish that wish. If I were a surrogate again that would be the last baby. I would know the couple I work with would have three children while I only had two."

Although she is occasionally curious about the baby she produced as a surrogate, Jane had no regrets as the child's first birthday approached. "I don't have any bitterness about the experience. I'm thankful I did what I did before the politicization of surrogacy," she said. She added that her surrogacy experience was interesting and worthwhile but that the births of her own two children stand out as the incredible moments of her life. "The surrogate child was the one who came and went. Her main impact on our lives is that my kids can now go to private school for two years. That's how the baby lives on for us."

The spring of 1987 found Elaine Silver swamped with phone calls—calls from the media in search of information about surrogate parenting, calls from prospective couples, and calls from prospective surrogates. The previous fall she had had so few clients that she had contemplated closing her New England center. The big change for her came in October when one of her surrogates—a woman who had recently delivered—volunteered her time and expertise to the center.

Elaine accepted her offer and set the woman to work screening phone calls and setting up appointments. This gave her more time to devote to screening couples and surrogates. And with the advent of the "Baby M" case Elaine readily admitted that screening had become far more important to her. If in the early years of her center she had been forced by demand to take on women whom society deemed undesirable candidates for surrogate mothers, after the "Baby M" case Elaine was no longer willing to take that risk. By the spring of 1987 she had begun to reject "inappropriate people—welfare mothers and women with possible criminal records, for example—without even seeing them in person. She had also drawn up a profile of what she considered to be an appropriate surrogate. According to Elaine, that woman "must be married or have an intact support system, and she can't be desperate for money."

Whatever happens with surrogate parenting in the future, Elaine hopes that courts nationwide will uphold surrogate parenting contracts. Unless that happens, she said, the "whole nature of surrogate parenting will be changed. The only security is in the contract. If you take that out there are no guarantees for couples or surrogates. I don't see the dust settling for ten years."

# Surrogate Parenting Clinics and Centers in the United States

(This is a listing of the major clinics open and operating at publication date that were willing to describe their programs.)

## California:

**CENTER FOR REPRODUCTIVE ALTERNATIVES**
3333 Vincent Road, Suite 222
Pleasant Hill, CA 94523

Bruce Rappaport, Ph.D., executive director; Marty Sochet, M.S.C.C., clinical director; Lyn Brown, administrative coordinator.
Established 1984.

Three employees. Refers to an obstetrician/gynecologist. Accepts 3 to 5 couples a year, 30 surrogates.

Psychological and medical testing required for surrogates and couples. No credit checks.

Meeting between couples and surrogates required. Location of artificial insemination procedures is determined by the individual surrogates and couple with a physician of their choice.

Fees—$25,000 to $30,000 overall. Details worked out in individual contracts.

Clinic may maintain contact with couples or surrogates indefinitely.

**CENTER FOR REPRODUCTIVE ALTERNATIVES**
727 Via Otono
San Clemente, CA 92672

Kathryn Wyckoff, director and sole staff member. Holds a degree in education. Established in Ohio in 1981. Moved facilities to San Clemente in July 1984.

Refers to a psychologist, a physician, several lawyers, and a parenting resource service. Accepts about 15 couples and 15 surrogates annually. Never handles more than 10 cases at a time.

Personal consultations required for surrogates and couples along with psychological screening. Medical screening for couples and surrogates includes tests for AIDS and herpes. No credit checks or checks of criminal records.

Contact between couples and surrogates encouraged but not mandatory. Both fresh and frozen semen used for artificial insemination. Insemination conducted either by a physician recommended by the clinic or by a physician chosen by the couple and the surrogate.

Fees—$18,000+ overall: $6,000 for the surrogate and $12,000 to the clinic, with the couple providing an additional $75 a month to the surrogate for the duration of the pregnancy for "out of pocket" expenses.

Clinic may maintain contact with couples or surrogates indefinitely.

**HAGAR INSTITUTE, SAN FRANCISCO FRANCHISE**
401 Marina Blvd.
Suite 125
San Francisco, CA 94080

Beth Bacon, director.
Established 1986.

Two employees. Refers to psychologists and physicians.

Accepted one couple and one surrogate in 1986. Expects to increase this number.

Psychological, social, genetic, and medical evaluation required.

Screening for criminal tendencies during psychological exam. No credit checks.

Contact between couples and surrogates encouraged though not mandatory. Insemination usually takes place at surrogate's discretion. Fresh semen preferred.

Fees—about $20,000 overall. Surrogate fee is $10,000, clinic fee is $9,500 plus $500 for a home study.

Intensive contact with surrogates and couples maintained for one month after the birth, after which contact is maintained at the discretion of the individual.

**WILLIAM W. HANDEL, J.D., LAW OFFICES**
8383 Wilshire Blvd.
Suite 750
Beverly Hills, CA 90211
(Also known as the Center of Surrogate Parenting)

William Handel, director; Hilary Hanafin, staff psychologist.

Established in 1980 as part of the then Sherwyn and Handel law office. In 1986 the partnership dissolved and Handel formed the Center of Surrogate Parenting.

Seven full-time staff members, including Handel and Hanafin. Referrals to fertility experts. Caroline O'Connell Public Relations handles publicity.

Accepts 30 couples a year and 60 surrogates. Maintains a caseload of 40.

Psychological screening conducted on premises for couples and surrogates. Test includes screening for criminality. Surrogates required to attend a support group. Outside fertility experts conduct physicals. No credit checks.

Contact between couples and surrogates is required. Artificial insemination in the Los Angeles area with clinic referred fertility experts preferred. Father may ship frozen semen.

Fees—$18,000+ overall; surrogate fee is $9,000 plus all

expenses, including maternity clothes, life insurance, transportation, child care and pregnancy-related supplies. Clinic fee is $9,000.

The legal department maintains contact with both surrogates and couples for a year and a half, the psychologist for a year, and both parties are asked to inform the center of address changes for 18 years following the birth of the baby.

## THE SURROGATE PARENT PROGRAM
11110 Ohio Ave.
Suite 202
Los Angeles, CA 90025

Nina Kellogg, Ph.D., director and sole member.
Fertility counseling since 1977. Surrogate parenting clinic established in 1981.

Refers to lawyers and physicians.
Maintains a caseload of at least 10 surrogates and couples annually.

Kellogg personally screens all surrogates and couples, conducting a one-time, controlled meeting between both parties and ongoing group counseling for surrogates. No credit checks.

At least one meeting between a couple and surrogate is required. Artificial insemination conducted at doctor's office of the clinic's choice or at offices of recommended physicians.

Fees—approximately $20,000 overall. Surrogate receives between $5,000 and $10,000.

Contact with clinic maintained as desired.

## BERNARD SHERWYN, J.D.
10880 Wilshire Blvd.
Suite 614
Los Angeles, CA 90024

(Also known as Surrogate Parenting Professionals.)
Bernard Sherwyn, director.
Established 1986.

Four employees. Refers to physicians and psychologists. Handles most legal work personally. Surrogates seek separate counsel.

Accepts about 12 couples and 15 surrogates a year. Maintains caseload of 10.

Psychological, medical testing—including AIDS and herpes—required for both surrogates and couples. Some genetic screening for surrogates. Emphasis on face-to-face interviewing. No credit or criminal checks.

Meeting between surrogate and couple required. May work on a first-name basis only. Only limited contact encouraged. Insemination takes place in the office of a clinic-designated physician. Use of fresh semen is encouraged but not mandatory.

Fees—about $22,000 to $25,000 overall. Clinic fee is $10,000 and surrogate fee is $12,000 plus $75 a month for expenses.

Keeps informal contact with both surrogate and couple two months after birth. Asks both parties to keep the clinic abreast of address changes for the child's first 18 years.

## Kansas:

HAGAR INSTITUTE
1015 Buchanan
Topeka, KS 66604

Beth Bacon, director.
Established 1982.

Five full-time and three part-time employee. Refers to psychologists and physicians.

Accepts 40 couples and 40 surrogates annually.

Social study, psychological exam, reference check, genetic screening required for surrogates and couples with attention paid during sessions to possible criminal record. Surrogates also undergo gynecological examination. No credit checks.

Contact between surrogates and couples is encouraged though not mandatory. Insemination generally scheduled in the office of a physician of the surrogate's choice. Fresh semen preferred but not required.

Fees—overall fee is $18,500; surrogate fee is $8,500; clinic fee is $9,500 plus $500 for a home study.

Intensive contact maintained with both surrogate and couple for one month after birth. Clinic may maintain contact indefinitely after that period.

## Kentucky:

**SURROGATE FAMILY SERVICES INC.**
713 West Main St.
Louisville, KY 40202

Katie Brophy, J.D., director.
Drafted first surrogate parenting contract in Kentucky in conjunction with Dr. Richard Levin of Surrogate Parenting Associates in 1979.
Established this service in December of 1980.

Three full-time employees. Refers to physicians and psychologists. Legal work handled in-house.

Accepts 12 to 15 surrogates and couples annually.

Physical and psychological exams required for surrogates,

medical exams for fathers. Surrogates may stipulate further testing for fathers as well. Couples may request background checks on surrogates, including criminal record. Couples determine how much contact they will have with surrogates. No specific location for insemination required. Fresh and frozen semen accepted. Fees—clinic fee is about $8,000. Couples and surrogates negotiate surrogate fee. The clinic maintains contact following the birth to the extent both surrogate and couples desire.

**SURROGATE PARENTING ASSOCIATES**
Suite 222
Doctor's Office Building
250 East Liberty St.
Louisville, KY 40202

Dr. Richard Levin, director, reproductive endrogrinologist. Established 1979.

Two full-time employees with assistance from medical office staff. Does some referring.

Receives about 400 inquiries annually from prospective surrogates and couples. Accepts all couples who can afford the process and are verifiably infertile and a commensurate number of surrogates. Would not specify.

Medical history, physical, and genetic study required for surrogates, along with a psychological exam, including VD and AIDS screening for the father. No screening for couples. No credit checks or specific checks for criminal records.

Strict anonymity maintained. Artificial insemination conducted in Levin's office. Fresh or frozen semen accepted.

Fees—about $20,000+ overall; surrogate fee is $10,000 to $12,000; clinic fee is $7,000 plus unspecified expenses. Clinic may maintain contact with both parties indefinitely.

# Maryland:

**INFERTILITY ASSOCIATES**
5530 Wisconsin Ave.
Chevy Chase, MD 20815

Harriet Blankfield, director.
Established in 1980 as the National Center for Surrogate Parenting. Name changed in 1985 to Infertility Associates.

Three full-time employees. Refers to physicians and other professionals as needed.

Accepts about 100 couples and 125 surrogates annually. Couples must be certifiably infertile. Prospective fathers tested for hepatitis B, herpes, AIDS and required to undergo a brief sperm analysis, as well as psychological assessment. Prenatal, medical, and psychological exams required for surrogates, who undergo similar disease testing as the father.

Strict anonymity maintained. Artificial insemination takes place at the office of a physician of the clinic's choice. As only fresh semen is used, the father must be present.

Fees—ranges from $20,000 to $30,00 overall; one-time agency fee is $12,000; surrogate fee is $10,000 plus up to $8,000 in expenses.

Clinic maintains contact with surrogates and couples at least six months following the birth. May stay in touch indefinitely.

# Massachusetts:

**NEW ENGLAND SURROGATE PARENTING PROGRAM**
130 Maple St.
Springfield, MA 01103

Laraine Shore-Suslowitz, director, clinical social worker.

Two full-time employees. Refers to physicians, fertility experts, and lawyers. Handles counseling in-house.

Accepts as many couples and surrogates annually as can be handled. Maintains caseload of 5 to 10.

Interviews required for the couple, along with sperm analysis for the father. Psychological and medical exams required for the surrogate. No credit or criminal checks.

Contact between surrogate and couple encouraged though may communicate on a first-name basis only or via the clinic. Only fresh sperm used for artificial insemination. Inseminations arranged at the office of a physician of the clinic's choice.

Fees—$20,000 to $30,000 overall; clinic fee is $10,000; surrogate fee is $10,000 plus any expenses negotiated with the couple prior to signing a contract.

Clinic may maintain contact with surrogates and couples indefinitely.


## Michigan:


**NOEL KEANE**
930 Mason
Dearborn, MI 48124
Established 1976 as an adjunct to Keane's law practice.

Employs 2 full-time lawyers and 6 secretaries. Refers to medical and psychological specialists.

Accepts about 200 couples and 450 surrogates annually.

Disease testing required for the father. Surrogates must submit to psychological and medical exams. Legal work handled by the law practice. No criminal screening.

No information available on anonymity. Fresh and frozen semen accepted for insemination. Insemination takes place at the office of a physician of the clinic or surrogate's choice. Fees—about $20,000 overall; clinic fee is $10,000; surrogate fee is $10,000.

No information on contact with surrogates or couples after birth.

## New York:

**INFERTILITY CENTER OF NEW YORK**
14 East 60th St.
Suite 1204
New York, NY 10022

Noel Keane, J.D., director.
Established in 1983 as an adjunct to Keane's Michigan center.

Keane supervises an administrator and two secretaries. Refers to medical and psychological specialists.

Accepts about 200 couples a year and 225 surrogates.

Screening requirements and artificial insemination procedures the same as the Michigan operation.

Fees—same as Michigan operation.

No information available on how much long-term contact is maintained.

**THE SURROGATE MOTHER PROGRAM**
640 West End Ave.
Apt. 3D
New York, NY 10024

Betsy Aigen, Psy.D., director.
Established 1984.

Four full-time employees. Refers to her husband, Isadore Schmukler, Ph.D., for psychological assessments of surrogates and research on surrogate behavior; and to physicians for physical examinations and inseminations, fertility specialists, gynecologists, insurance agents, and lawyers. In the process of establishing a sperm bank, radiology and laboratory facilities and offices for on-site inseminations.

Maintains a caseload of 20 couples. Accepts 50 surrogates into the program annually.

Extensive psychological screening required for both couples and surrogates. Couples should expect questioning on their marriage and past medical history. Husband required to submit to complete physical, including tests for AIDS, herpes, and VD. Surrogates' psychological testing includes environmental and sociological checks, emotional, genetic, and historical screening, screening of all immediate family members, prenatal lab screening, fertility screening when required, and complete physical, including screening for AIDS, herpes, and VD. No criminal or credit checks.

Couples and surrogates determine how much contact is preferable. Clinic encourages contact. Fresh and frozen semen accepted for artificial insemination. Clinic prefers insemination to take place on the premises but will make exceptions.

Fees—$22,000 to $25,000 overall; surrogate fee is $10,000; clinic fee is $8,500. Attorney fees, physical exams, insemination fees, psychological testing, genetic screening, life and medical insurance for surrogate, maternity clothes, adoption fees, paternity tests, mail, telephone, travel and postpartum counseling all extra.

Clinic contacts all surrogates one year after the birth of the child and asks surrogates to maintain contact with the clinic for 18 years following the birth. Some couples are asked to be involved in follow-up studies. May maintain contact with all couples indefinitely.

## Oregon:

**SURROGATE FOUNDATION**
P.O. Box 06545
Portland, OR 97206

Norma Thorsen, director.
Established in 1983 as a "service organization."

Ms. Thorsen is sole staff member. Refers to physicians, psychologists, and lawyers.

Accepts about 7 couples and 20 surrogates annually.

Sperm analysis required for father, along with complete physical.

Testing for AIDS also required. Psychological exam and genetic history required for couple. Physical, gynecological, and psychological exams required for surrogate. No criminal checks.

Contact between couples and surrogates not encouraged though permitted. Fresh and frozen semen accepted for artificial insemination. Insemination at the office of a physician of surrogate's choice.

Fees—about $18,000 overall. Foundation fee is $6,000; surrogate fee is $10,000 to $12,000 depending on agreed-upon expenses.

Maintains contact with both surrogates and couples for at least six weeks after the birth.

# Questions Couples and Surrogates Ask Most Often When Considering Surrogate Parenting:

### How to find a clinic or center?

Most advertise in large-city newspapers and alternative papers such as *The Village Voice.*

Check with local fertility specialists or gynecologists.

Check the library or your local newspaper for clippings about clinics that have opened in your area.

### How to choose a clinic or center?

Analyze your personal style. Do you like things to be highly businesslike?

Relaxed? Personal or impersonal?

There are clinics that meet just about any personal taste.

Be aware of varying clinic policies on insemination, anonymity, fees, and ways of handling the birth.

Choose the clinic that offers the amount of contact you prefer to maintain with a surrogate or couple.

Be aware that screening policies differ from one clinic to another. Choose the amount of screening that makes you feel confident and secure in your choice of surrogate or couple.

Look for clinics with support groups. Psychologists believe these groups help both surrogates and couples cope with the surrogacy process.

## What should you expect during the surrogacy process?

Be prepared for extensive background probing, psychological and medical examinations.

Be prepared to deal with outside specialists, including lawyers, psychologists, physicians, and fertility experts.

Be prepared to meet your surrogate or couple at least once.

Be prepared to travel for the artificial insemination unless your clinic of choice works with frozen semen.

Be prepared as a couple to spend at least $15,000. Surrogates can expect to earn about $10,000 plus expenses. (Note that costs generally exceed the base fees. Be sure to spell out all differences up front.)

Be prepared to meet your surrogate or couple in the hospital at the time of birth.

Be aware that relinquishment proceedings usually take place in the hospital following the birth. In most states, adoption does not take place until six months later.

Be prepared to maintain contact with the clinic for up to 18 years following the birth. Many clinics are now doing follow-up research on surrogates or couples, or keep updated records.

# INDEX

132-33, 155, 169-70,
180

Hagar Institute, Kansas and
Cal., 163, 164, 167, 172-73,
177, 179, 206-7, 209-10
Hanafin, Hilary, 85-89, 134-41,
172, 178, 181, 207
Handel, William W., 164, 181,
207
Harrison, Dennis Michael, 94,
95
Hospitals, and surrogate birth,
32, 174

Impotency, fear of, 59-60, 85
Infertility
and resource allocation,
189-90
of surrogate couples, 39-
40, 43-44, 46, 85, 86-87,
90, 148-49, 150-51, 156-
57
Infertility Associates, Md., 164,
169, 212
Infertility Center of New York,
164, 214
Insemination process, 59-60,
62-65, 85, 90, 106-7
with fresh vs frozen
semen, 170-71
In vitro fertilization, 81, 189

Johnson, Laurie, 122-23, 131

Kansas, 177, 209-10
Keane, Noel, 82, 120, 161, 164,
168, 176, 177, 179-80, 213,
214

Kentucky, 176, 210-11

Levin, Richard, 164, 211

McKnight, Becky, 127
McRobbie, Bernard Glennon,
20, 71, 199
McRobbie, Glenn and Linda,
11-13, 15, 20-77, 199-202
Martin, Nancy and Carl, 82, 93,
94-95, 98
Maryland, 212
Massachusetts, 12, 26, 27, 105,
212-13
Michigan, 176, 213-14
Mothers. *See* Adoptive moth-
ers; Surrogate mothers

National Association of Surrogate Mothers, 123, 125, 130-
31
National Committee for Adoption, 14
*New Conceptions* (Andrews),
12, 162, 176
New England Surrogate Parenting Program, Mass., 212-
13
New York State, 26, 214-16

Ohio, 176-77
Oregon, 216

Parker, Philip, 120, 168
Pierce, William, 14

Rappaport, Bruce, 89

Schmukler, Isadore, 121, 130,